A Clinician's Guide to Using Light Therapy

A Clinician's Guide to Using Light Therapy

RAYMOND W. LAM, MD, FRCPC

Professor and Head of the Mood and Anxiety Disorders Program in the Department of Psychiatry, University of British Columbia, and Director of the Mood Disorders Centre of Excellence at UBC Hospital, Vancouver, Canada.

EDWIN M. TAM, MDCM, FRCPC

Clinical Associate Professor at the Department of Psychiatry, University of British Columbia, and UBC Hospital, Vancouver, Canada.

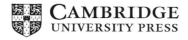

CAMBRIDGE
UNIVERSITY PRESS

CAMBRIDGE
UNIVERSITY PRESS

University Printing House, Cambridge CB2 8BS, United Kingdom

One Liberty Plaza, 20th Floor, New York, NY 10006, USA

477 Williamstown Road, Port Melbourne, VIC 3207, Australia

314-321, 3rd Floor, Plot 3, Splendor Forum, Jasola District Centre, New Delhi - 110025, India

79 Anson Road, #06-04/06, Singapore 079906

Cambridge University Press is part of the University of Cambridge.

It furthers the University's mission by disseminating knowledge in the pursuit of education, learning and research at the highest international levels of excellence.

www.cambridge.org
Information on this title: www.cambridge.org/9780521697682

First published 2009

A catalogue record for this publication is available from the British Library

Library of Congress Cataloging in Publication data
Lam, Raymond W., 1956–
    A clinician's guide to using light therapy / Raymond W. Lam, Edwin M. Tam.
        p. ; cm.
    Includes bibliographical references and index.
    ISBN 978-0-521-69768-2 (pbk.)
    1. Seasonal affective disorder–Treatment.   2. Phototherapy.   I. Tam, Edwin M.   II. Title.
    [DNLM: 1. Seasonal Affective Disorder–therapy.   2. Phototherapy–methods.
    WM 171 L213c 2009]
    RC545.L36 2009
    616.85´27–dc22
    2009027556

ISBN 978-0-521-69768-2 Paperback

CONTENTS

Contents

Contents

Preface

- Light as therapy
- How to use this book
- Abbreviations used

Light as therapy

Light is ever-present in our daily lives. We experience light as the gentle arrival of dawn, the first flip of a room light switch, the warmth of the noonday sun, the glorious colours of the sunset, and the cool beams of moonlight. Light is represented in everyday expressions of speech and as scenes and symbols in literature and the media in every culture throughout the ages.

Given its ubiquitous presence, perhaps it is not so surprising that light would have healing properties. We have been studying and treating people with light for the past 20 years. We began as skeptics and first designed and conducted controlled studies to convince ourselves that light therapy was not just an elaborate placebo. We have been gratified to see the rapid responses that people experience with light therapy and the difference it has made to the lives of so many. We expected that this effective non-pharmacological treatment that made so much sense would be enthusiastically embraced by physicians and mental health clinicians everywhere.

Unfortunately, there are wide chasms between scientific evidence and clinical adoption. Despite its simplicity and effectiveness, light therapy was not widely used. Although disappointed, at first we understood the poor clinical uptake: the original light boxes were large, expensive, and difficult to obtain, and the lower intensities they produced required two to four hours of daily exposure. With all these limitations, light treatment was used only by the most motivated people. But when light devices became more portable, more affordable, and more easily purchased, and when the duration of treatment was reduced to only 30 minutes a day, we expected that light therapy would take off. In 1999 we published clinical guidelines for clinicians to follow when using this excellent treatment. We waited eagerly for light therapy to become widely available in clinical settings.

Not so. Again, we were disappointed. The uptake for light therapy continued to be slow, despite the popular and successful courses that we gave at major psychiatric and professional conferences. It was clear that clinical adoption of new non-pharmacological treatments was very challenging for both physicians (psychiatrists and family doctors) and for mental health professionals. They needed more guidance about the practical details of using light therapy than scientific articles or textbooks could provide.

That observation was the inspiration for writing this book. It is not a reference textbook or a systematic scientific review. Rather, we have drawn on our collective 35 years of clinical and scientific experience to provide a simple, step-by-step guide to prescribe light therapy and to incorporate its use within a busy clinical practice. We hope that this practical book will help to make light therapy accessible to many more clinicians and to the patients that they treat.

How to use this book

Because light therapy is used primarily for treating seasonal affective disorder (SAD), we begin in Chapter 1 by providing some "tips and traps" for recognizing, diagnosing, and assessing SAD and other related conditions. Those readers who are experienced in diagnosis can go immediately to Chapter 2, which describes a simple method for using light treatment. Chapter 3 covers the practical aspects of evaluating and purchasing light devices. Other treatments for SAD, which can be used alone or combined with light, are described in Chapter 4. We left the summary of scientific evidence for the effectiveness of light therapy and theories about its mechanism(s) of action for Chapter 5. In Chapter 6, we briefly review some of the other conditions (both seasonal and nonseasonal) in which light has been studied and in which it can be used clinically, along with practical considerations of how the light treatment method is modified. Finally, Chapter 7 provides many clinician resources that are helpful for using light therapy. The rating scales and patient handouts can be photocopied for clinical use and masters are also available for free download at our website, www.UBCsad.ca. This book is not extensively referenced like a scientific paper or a textbook. Instead, we provide a "Further reading" section at the end of each chapter with major references in the field and a list of reference books in Chapter 7.

We dedicate this book to our research mentors, Dr. J. Christian Gillin (in memoriam) and Dr. Daniel F. Kripke at the University of California,

San Diego, whose sage scientific and professional advice has always been welcome, and to all our colleagues and patients (past, present and future) at the Seasonal Mood Disorders Clinic at UBC Hospital.

Abbreviations used

5-HIAA	5-hydroxyindoleacetic acid
5-HT	5-hydroxytryptamine (serotonin)
ADHD	Attention deficit hyperactivity disorder
CBT	Cognitive behavioural therapy
DLMO	Dim light melatonin onset
DSM-IV	Diagnostic and Statistical Manual of Mental Disorders, 4th Edition
DSPS	Delayed sleep phase syndrome
EEG	Electroencephalography
Ham-D	Hamilton Depression Rating Scale
LED	Light-emitting diode
MDD	Major depressive disorder
MDE	Major depressive episodes
MEQ	Morningness-Eveningness Questionnaire
MT	Melatonin receptor
PHQ-9	Patient Health Questionnaire, 9-item version
PIDS	Personal Inventory of Depression and Seasonality
PMDD	Premenstrual dysphoric disorder
QIDS-SR	Quick Inventory of Depressive Symptomatology, Self-Rated
RCT	Randomized controlled trial
SAD	Seasonal affective disorder
SCN	Suprachiasmatic nucleus
SIGH-SAD	Structured Interview Guide for the Ham-D, SAD version
SPAQ	Seasonal Pattern Assessment Questionnaire
SSRI	Selective serotonin reuptake inhibitor
STAR*D	Sequenced Treatment Alternatives to Relieve Depression study

1

Seasonal Affective Disorder: Diagnostic Issues

- Definition and diagnostic criteria
- Prevalence and burden
- Screening
- Clinical features
- Differential diagnosis
- Variants of SAD
- Further reading

Definition and diagnostic criteria

Seasonal affective disorder (SAD), otherwise known as winter depression, was first systematically described by Dr. Norman Rosenthal and colleagues in their classic 1984 paper describing SAD and its treatment with light therapy. SAD was conceptualized as a type of depression with recurrent winter depressive episodes (which included both major and minor depressive episodes, although at least one had to be major) and full remission of symptoms (or a switch into hypomania or mania, if bipolar) in the spring and summer.

Since then, the diagnostic criteria for SAD have undergone revision in various diagnostic systems leading up to the DSM-IV (the prevailing diagnostic manual used in psychiatry). In DSM-IV, SAD is not listed as a separate diagnosis but instead is defined as a subtype of depression with recurrent major depressive episodes (MDEs, Table 1.1). In summary, an MDE consists of at least two weeks of either pervasive (during most of the day, on most days) low mood or significantly reduced ability to experience pleasure (anhedonia), in conjunction with a cluster of at least five of nine characteristic symptoms. These symptoms must cause significant distress and/or seriously affect function at work, home, or with others. Finally, other causes of depressive symptoms, including bereavement, medical conditions, medication side effects and substance abuse, must be ruled out.

Diagnostic Tip

People are sometimes loath to describe themselves as "depressed". Some may have specific associations with the word "depressed" that make it seem like an inaccurate description ("My mother was in bed all day with depression: I'm not like that"). Others may have fears of being labeled, appearing weak, or being stigmatized. There are many descriptors for feeling depressed (blue, low, down, empty, melancholy, blah, etc.) and it may be useful to ask about these should "sadness" be initially denied.

Some people describe low interest and enjoyment as feeling "bored" or "apathetic". Low interest is often masked by related symptoms of low energy or motivation, which can also reduce participation in pleasurable activities. Asking about enjoyment of passive activities that do not require effort, such as listening to music or watching television, may differentiate interest from activity level.

Table 1.1.   **DSM-IV criteria for major depressive episode (MDE).**

A Five (or more) of the following symptoms have been present during the same 2-week period and represent a change from previous functioning; at least one of the symptoms is either (1) depressed mood or (2) loss of interest or pleasure. **Note:** Do not include symptoms that are clearly due to a general medical condition, or mood-incongruent delusions or hallucinations.

   (1) depressed mood most of the day, nearly every day, as indicated by either subjective report (e.g., feels sad or empty) or observation made by others (e.g., appears tearful). **Note:** In children and adolescents, can be irritable mood

   (2) markedly diminished interest or pleasure in all, or almost all, activities most of the day, nearly every day (as indicated by either subjective account or observation made by others);

   (3) significant weight loss when not dieting or weight gain (e.g., a change of more than 5% of body weight in a month), or decrease or increase in appetite nearly every day. **Note:** In children, consider failure to make expected weight gains

   (4) insomnia or hypersomnia nearly every day

   (5) psychomotor agitation or retardation nearly every day (observable by others, not merely subjective feelings of restlessness or being slowed down)

   (6) fatigue or loss of energy nearly every day

   (7) feelings of worthlessness or excessive or inappropriate guilt (which may be delusional) nearly every day (not merely self-reproach or guilt about being sick)

   (8) diminished ability to think or concentrate, or indecisiveness, nearly every day (either by subjective account or as observed by others)

Table 1.1.	(cont.)

(9) recurrent thoughts of death (not just fear of dying), recurrent suicidal ideation without a specific plan, or a suicide attempt or a specific plan for committing suicide

B The symptoms do not meet criteria for a Mixed Episode.

C The symptoms cause clinically significant distress or impairment in social, occupational, or other important areas of functioning.

D The symptoms are not due to the direct physiological effects of a substance (e.g., a drug of abuse, a medication) or a general medical condition (e.g., hypothyroidism).

E The symptoms are not better accounted for by bereavement, i.e., after the loss of a loved one, the symptoms persist for longer than 2 months or are characterized by marked functional impairment, morbid preoccupation with worthlessness, suicidal ideation, psychotic symptoms, or psychomotor retardation.

DSM-IV categorizes subtypes of MDEs as episode specifiers (based on the cross-sectional symptoms during an episode) and as course specifiers (based on the pattern of depressive episodes) (Table 1.2). The "With Seasonal Pattern" specifier, equivalent to SAD, can apply to both unipolar major depressive disorder (MDD) and to bipolar disorder (either Type I – with manic episodes, or Type II – with hypomanic episodes). Although the pattern of seasonal episodes is not specified, the overwhelming majority of people with seasonal pattern suffer from fall/winter depressions. From now on, when referring to SAD, we mean the DSM-IV definition of recurrent MDD with a seasonal winter pattern.

Making a diagnosis of SAD can be challenging because it is based on recognizing and characterizing of depressive episodes that go back many years. Table 1.3 lists the DSM-IV criteria for seasonal pattern. Some of these criteria are evidence-based, while others are more controversial. And, while the criteria may seem straightforward, the clinical presentation may be more difficult. We will illustrate some key diagnostic issues as we examine each criterion in more detail.

Table 1.2.	DSM-IV specifiers for major depressive episodes.

Episode specifiers	Course specifiers
• With melancholic features (non-reactive mood, anhedonia, weight loss, guilt, psychomotor retardation or agitation, morning worsening of mood, early morning awakening) • With atypical features (reactive mood, oversleeping, overeating, leaden paralysis, interpersonal rejection sensitivity) • With psychotic features (hallucinations and/or delusions) • With catatonic features (motor signs and symptoms, uncommonly seen in clinical practice)	• With seasonal pattern (equivalent to seasonal affective disorder) • With postpartum onset (within 1 month of delivery) • With rapid cycling (more than four episodes in one year, applies to bipolar disorder)

Table 1.3.	DSM-IV criteria for seasonal pattern specifier.

Episode specifier

With Seasonal Pattern (can be applied to the pattern of Major Depressive Episodes in Bipolar I Disorder, Bipolar II Disorder, or Major Depressive Disorder, Recurrent)

A There has been a regular temporal relationship between the onset of Major Depressive Episodes in Bipolar I or Bipolar II Disorder or Major Depressive Disorder, Recurrent, and a particular time of the year (e.g., regular appearance of the Major Depressive Episode in the fall or winter). Note: Do not include cases in which there is an obvious effect of seasonal-related psychosocial stressors (e.g., regularly being unemployed every winter).

B Full remissions (or a change from depression to mania or hypomania) also occur at a characteristic time of the year (e.g., depression disappears in the spring).

C In the last 2 years, two Major Depressive Episodes have occurred that demonstrate the temporal seasonal relationships defined in Criteria A and B, and no nonseasonal Major Depressive Episodes have occurred during that same period.

D Seasonal Major Depressive Episodes (as described above) substantially outnumber the nonseasonal Major Depressive Episodes that may have occurred over the individual's lifetime.

Regular time of onset

Onset of an episode is very difficult to pinpoint, in part because symptoms often come on gradually. Additionally, even in people with well-established SAD, the episode onset can vary from year to year, depending on factors such as weather patterns and life stresses. Practically, patients can usually specify regular onset within a given month, e.g., October or November. We also find it useful to ask about the month when symptoms are typically at their worst (in our clinical samples, usually January), because treatment may need to be adjusted during this time. Note that SAD also occurs in the southern hemisphere, where the winter months are opposite to those in Canada!

Not due to seasonal stressor

While it may be intuitive to exclude depressive symptoms caused by regularly occurring seasonal stressors, in practice this can be difficult to determine. For example, many occupations have stressors with a seasonal component, which then requires clinical judgment as to whether all symptoms can be attributed to the seasonal stressor.

Clinical example

Robert is a retired man who reports recent onset of depressions during the last few winters. On examination, his low mood was associated with his friends leaving town each winter for vacations, which he could not join because of financial reasons. Likewise, relief of symptoms was more connected to their time of return than to any particular time of year. He himself stated that the loneliness was the major factor in his depression. He was therefore not diagnosed with SAD.

Some patients may not have a clear idea themselves about the relationship between seasonal stressors and depressive symptoms. Consider the common scenario of a college student, where return to school coincides with the fall season onset of depressive symptoms. Are the SAD symptoms simply due to academic stresses? A careful history may reveal that the symptoms are independent of stress.

Clinical example

Vicky is a college student who experiences onset of depressive symptoms in the fall, coincident with October midterm exams. However, a careful history reveals that the symptoms start in early October, well before the exam period. Also, she had faced exam stresses in the spring/summer without experiencing similar symptoms. Based on these findings, Vicky's symptoms were attributed to SAD.

Full remissions in the spring/summer

Just as there is variability in onset time, so can there be variability in offset time. Again, patients usually are able to recall the month when they are feeling back to their usual selves. A more difficult distinction is whether a switch into hypomania occurs, because patients often do not view this as abnormal (see "Differential diagnosis"). Other patients will also report full remission in the summer, but on prospective monitoring will have residual depressive symptoms (see "Variants of SAD"). To detect these situations, it is very useful to have a summer assessment.

Clinical example

Ethan describes clear episodes of winter major depression with normal mood in the summer, thus meeting criteria for SAD. After successful winter treatment with light therapy, he was assessed the following summer. He noted that he did not feel as well as he remembered, especially on cloudy days, and still had many symptoms of depression. The summer reassessment showed that Ethan had a more chronic and nonseasonal course of depression than he realized.

SAD episodes in last two years and no nonseasonal episodes

The rationale for including this criterion was to ensure that the seasonal pattern is an active clinical issue and not just a past condition. By limiting to the last two episodes, the intent was to reduce recall bias, since recent symptoms and course are more likely to be accurately remembered.

Unfortunately, there is no evidence to support the validity or necessity of this criterion. The pattern of episodes for patients with SAD can vary and sometimes patients will "skip" a winter episode or have a longer-than-usual episode (i.e. extending into spring and summer). This may be due to external factors, such as weather conditions (e.g., an uncommonly dark and cloudy spring), a significant life stressor (e.g., break-up of a relationship in the summer), the use of antidepressant medications, or living in more southerly latitudes.

Clinical example

Roger had a regular pattern of winter MDEs for four consecutive past years. He started using bupropion, with effect, and continued using the medication without an episode the following winter. He then discontinued the bupropion in the summer because he wanted to try light therapy the next winter. He had his usual onset of depressive symptoms in November and met criteria for an MDE. However, he no longer met DSM-IV criteria for seasonal pattern because he did not have an episode last year when he was taking bupropion. In Roger's case, the use of antidepressants masked the regular winter pattern of episodes.

Vicky had a clear pattern of SAD when she lived in Toronto, but then moved to Phoenix to study for a year. During the sunny winter in Phoenix, she did not experience any symptoms. However, on return to Toronto the following year Vicky again had characteristic symptoms in the winter – but she no longer met DSM-IV criteria for SAD because of her time in Arizona.

In summary, examining the overall clinical picture is more informative than restricting to the last two years. Given the controversy over this issue, even among specialists in the field, we support allowing clinical judgment to over-ride this criterion when appropriate. We tend be more stringent in applying the "two-year rule" to patients with new-onset SAD who were previously untreated.

Seasonal substantially outnumber nonseasonal episodes

Previous versions of the DSM used a ratio of 3:1 for seasonal to nonseasonal episodes, but again there are no data for this criterion. Consequently, DSM-IV is purposely vague about the definition for "substantially outnumber" and it remains within clinical judgment. For someone with several previous nonseasonal depressions, we tend to put more weight on the pattern of recent episodes.

Other diagnostic tips and traps

Accuracy is always an issue when dealing with retrospective recall. Short of keeping a journal, few people self-monitor to the point of tracking all the symptoms of depression over the course of each episode. Sometimes people are overly enthusiastic about the diagnosis, in part because of its novelty or their desire for light therapy, which may lead them to mistakenly report seasonal episodes.

Clinical example

Dolores reads a lot and is convinced that she suffers from SAD. However, her doctor of many years clearly documented her previous depressive episodes and a chart review shows no evidence of seasonal pattern. Further exploration revealed that she was disenchanted with medications and was hoping to use light therapy. While disappointed about not having SAD, Dolores was glad to find out that light therapy may also be helpful for nonseasonal depression.

Conversely, we have seen some skeptical patients who see only a chain of coincidences when confronted with a clear pattern of winter depressions. Careful charting of episodes, inspection of old charts and, if possible, collateral information from family members can help clarify seasonal patterns.

Clinical example

Ted is a man in his fifties who had been skeptical throughout his life of the idea of having a mental illness. However, in reviewing his life history, he couldn't help but notice that every relationship breakup that he had ever suffered had occurred in the fall months. Further history revealed untreated winter depressions over many years and a diagnosis of SAD was made.

Since patients usually present in the winter during a depressive episode, we find it simpler to first establish a diagnosis of MDE, since it is easier for patients to describe current signs and symptoms. Once the current episode is characterized, we turn our attention to establish regular onsets of previous depressive episodes, starting from the most recent and working backward. If the current episode is mild or equivocal, then it may be more productive to look back at the person's most severe depressive episode, or the one best remembered, in order to see whether it meets criteria for MDE. Finally, we check on summer symptoms and whether full remission occurs, and whether they have had hypomanic or manic episodes, or nonseasonal depressive episodes. Only with all this information can one make the diagnosis of SAD with confidence.

Prevalence and burden

The quality of studies on the epidemiology of SAD has varied widely. Many studies used self-report questionnaires (such as the Seasonal Pattern Assessment Questionnaire, SPAQ) which were designed as screening tools and not as diagnostic instruments, and/or examined specific populations (such as college students) that cannot be used to determine the prevalence of SAD in the general community.

In Canada, it is estimated that 1 in 35 people (up to 1 million in total) have SAD; in the United States, it is 1 in 200 (up to 1.5 million people). The "average" patient with SAD presenting for treatment is a 38-year-old married woman who has had 10 previous episodes of winter depression.

Studies using proper psychiatric interviews and diagnostic criteria have found that SAD affects between 0.5% and 3% of the general population in northern countries, making it a very common psychiatric condition. In outpatient psychiatric clinics, up to 15% of patients with recurrent depression will have a seasonal winter pattern, with women having 1.6-times the risk of men. A higher percentage of people (7.5% to 20% in North America) may suffer from a milder variant of SAD, appropriately labeled "subsyndromal SAD" and colloquially known as the "winter blues".

In questionnaire studies of SAD, which probably lump together SAD and subsyndromal SAD, there appear to be higher rates reported in North Americans (0.7–9.7%) compared to Europeans (1.3–3%) and Asians (0–0.9%). There is also some evidence for increasing rates of SAD with higher (e.g., more northerly) latitudes. The risk for SAD increases with age until the mid-50s, and then becomes less common in older age groups.

Although SAD is sometimes portrayed in the popular press (and reflected in the opinion of some clinicians) as a trivial condition, studies have shown that people with SAD have significant impairment in daily function in winter. Quality of life is also severely reduced, to the same extent as in nonseasonal depression.

Screening

In some settings it may be helpful to screen people for seasonal depression. This can be done simply with the SPAQ, a brief questionnaire that measures seasonality and is widely used to screen for SAD. As with most screening questionnaires, the SPAQ will "over-diagnose", in that many people identified as having SAD will actually have subsyndromal SAD on diagnostic assessment. On the other hand, the SPAQ rarely misses someone with a true diagnosis of SAD. The SPAQ and its scoring criteria are included in Chapter 7.

The Personal Inventory for Depression and Seasonality (PIDS) is another good screening tool for SAD. An on-line version is available free at the Center for Environmental Therapeutics website, *www.cet.org* . Also available at that website for purchase is a clinician package of useful assessment tools.

Clinical features

The formal DSM-IV diagnostic criteria for SAD are based only on the pattern of MDEs, but it is well recognized that patients with SAD also experience characteristic symptoms during a winter depressive episode. These include increased sleep, appetite and weight, and fatigue and low energy. The majority of clinic samples of SAD present with these clinical features (Table 1.4).

These are often called "atypical" depressive symptoms to distinguish them from the more common and "typical" symptoms (e.g., insomnia, decreased appetite, weight loss) seen in melancholic-type depression. However, atypical is a poor term because these symptoms are actually quite commonly seen in patients with nonseasonal depression as well. For example, up to 40% of depressed patients seen in outpatient clinics will have atypical features.

Increased appetite, carbohydrate craving and overeating

The increased appetite experienced by people with SAD is commonly accompanied by carbohydrate craving for starches and sweets. This leads to increased eating which, in conjunction with decreased activity and exercise, leads to increased weight during depressive episodes. The weight gain experienced during winter depressions is not trivial, ranging from 2 to 20 or more pounds. Although the resolution of symptoms in the spring

Table 1.4. Clinical features in patients with bipolar and unipolar SAD seen at the UBC Hospital Mood Disorders Centre. Adapted from Sohn and Lam, 2004.

	Unipolar SAD (n=785)	Bipolar SAD (n=50)[a]
Demographics		
% female	71%	72%
Age (years)	37.2 ± 10.6	38.9 ± 11.5
Atypical symptoms		
Hypersomnia	69%	66%
Increased appetite	59%	64%
Carbohydrate craving	63%	67%
Weight gain	53%	58%
Other symptoms		
Insomnia	21%	28%
Loss of appetite	24%	18%
Weight loss	12%	12%
Anxiety	87%	92%
Panic attacks	8%	10%
Suicide risk		
Suicidal thoughts	47%	50%
Past suicidal attempt	10%	10%
Past history		
Past psychiatric hospitalization	12%	28%[b]
Number of past seasonal (winter) depressive episodes	9.7 ± 8	9.0 ± 6.8
Number of past nonseasonal depressive episodes	0.8 ± 1.5	0.7 ± 1.9
Total number of depressive episodes	10.8 ± 8.1	10.6 ± 7.2
Family history		
Mood disorder in first-degree relatives	59%	57%
Alcoholism in first-degree relatives	42%	47%

[a] Bipolar I, n=11; bipolar II, n=39.
[b] *Statistically significant difference, p < 0.0001.*

and summer often results in return to normal appetite and losing the extra weight, the average weight of people with SAD rises with each successive episode.

> ### Clinical example
>
> Vicky described a definite seasonal fluctuation in her weight which was consistent year after year with 10–15 pound weight gain in the winter and subsequent weight loss in the summer. She noted that her summer wardrobe was 2 sizes smaller than her winter one! More recently, however, the weight loss in the summer failed to fully reverse the weight gain of the previous winter. The thought of a continued "ratchet" effect motivated her to seek treatment for SAD.

The increased eating can also present as, or progress to, binge-eating, in which large amounts of food are ingested over a short time followed by intense feelings of regret and self-loathing. These food-related symptoms have led to observation of an overlap between SAD and bulimia nervosa, an eating disorder characterized by binge-eating and purging. Up to 30% of women with bulimia nervosa experience seasonal mood changes as severe as in SAD, with worsening of bingeing and purging during the winter.

Hypersomnia

Self-reported hypersomnia (increased sleeping) is often present in SAD and can be described by patients as "sleeping too well". Furthermore, it can coexist with insomnia (e.g., poor sleep at night results in fatigue, sleepiness and napping during the day), so both symptoms should be assessed. While many patients with SAD describe sleeping 10 to 12 or more hours each night and spend a lot of time in bed, objective measurement of sleep in a sleep laboratory does not show that they actually sleep more hours. Instead, the "oversleeping" is better characterized as an increased need for sleep, rather than increased sleep hours *per se*. The sleep they do have is non-restorative, which makes them feel groggy and have great difficulty awakening in the morning. The difficulty arising and feeling totally awake is also termed "sleep inertia".

Clinical example

Roger presents with complaints of sleeping too much and difficulty arising in the morning. He often naps during the day as well. On closer examination, he also reports significant insomnia, waking frequently in the night and often laying awake for an hour or more. The insomnia makes him sleep later than usual and causes daytime sleepiness. He has both insomnia and hypersomnia, because the 10 total hours he sleeps in 24 hours (including naps) is more than usual.

Low energy and fatigue

These are the most common symptoms in SAD, and often are experienced as an "afternoon slump" pattern with intense fatigue and sleepiness in the afternoon that recovers somewhat towards the evening. An extreme form of low energy is called "leaden paralysis", which is described as a physical feeling of heaviness in the arms and legs, as if they were made of lead, or as a sensation of walking through water.

Suicidal ideas

Thoughts of suicide often accompany depression, and SAD is no exception (Table 1.4). Fortunately, suicide attempts and deaths are uncommon in patients with SAD. Regardless, all depressed patients should be assessed for suicidal thoughts and plans. Table 1.5 lists common risk factors for suicide, based on the features of the depressive episode and on demographic features.

Of interest is that suicidal ideation is less commonly found in SAD compared to nonseasonal MDD. The predictable episodes in SAD may explain this finding. Hopelessness is one of the strongest correlates of suicidal thoughts and plans. People with SAD know that they will improve

| Table 1.5. | Risk factors for suicide in MDD (unspecified seasonality). |

Related to episode	Related to demographics
• Current suicidal plans • Prior attempts • Severe depression • Hopelessness and guilt • Inpatient or recently discharged • Bipolarity • Mixed state (with agitation), dysphoric mania • Psychotic features • Comorbidity (anxiety, substance abuse, serious medical conditions)	• Male • Adolescent or elderly • Early onset of mood disorder • Personality disorder (especially Cluster B) • Family history of suicide • Adverse childhood experiences (trauma, illness, parental loss) • Adverse life circumstances (unemployment, social isolation) • Recent psychosocial stressor • Lack of supports

once spring arrives, so they generally feel less hopeless than people with nonseasonal depression, who never know how long their depression will last.

Family history and genetics

Family history studies have suggested that there is a genetic component to SAD. Twin studies show that seasonal variability of mood is heritable, with up to 50% of the variance in seasonality scores explainable by genetic factors. Several candidate genes involving serotonin have been studied in SAD, although results are inconsistent. Similarly, there is interesting preliminary evidence that clock genes (i.e. genes involved with the structure and function of the circadian pacemaker) may be involved with seasonal mood changes, if not specifically to SAD. There is also recent evidence that clock genes may be implicated in bipolar disorder. For example, mice that are genetically modified so they do not have a specific clock gene (in this case, also called CLOCK) display behaviours that are very similar to mania.

Children and adolescents

Winter depressive symptoms and SAD have also been described in children and adolescents. Many adults with SAD report that their winter symptoms began in their teenage years. It can be difficult to distinguish seasonal depression from school stress because the school year overlaps with the winter season. The depressive symptoms in children with SAD can also include distractibility and poor concentration, and there is interesting new research about the links between SAD and attention deficit hyperactivity disorder (ADHD). Light therapy has also been found to be effective in paediatric and adolescent samples with SAD.

Differential diagnosis

Medical conditions or substance use/abuse

Medical illnesses can present with depressive symptoms. Most textbooks have long lists of diseases that are associated with depression, but common ones include anemia and thyroid conditions. Most physicians would include some blood tests for patients with depression, such as a complete blood count and thyroid-stimulating hormone (TSH) to rule out these conditions. Other blood tests are only necessary if indicated by symptoms on history or abnormal signs on physical examination.

Similarly, a long list of prescription medications and drugs of abuse are associated with depressive symptoms with regular use, intoxication or withdrawal. Again, common drugs associated with depression include alcohol and methamphetamine, so inquiring about substance use is important.

Bipolar disorder

Initial studies suggested that almost all patients with SAD could be diagnosed as having bipolar disorder. In part, this was due to liberal criteria for the diagnosis of hypomania in earlier diagnostic interviews. Since many people experience mood elevation in the spring, the contrast between recovering from depression and the spring "hyperthymic" state led to overdiagnosis of hypomania.

Subsequent studies using DSM criteria for mania and hypomania found that a smaller percentage, 11% to 19%, of patients with SAD have a bipolar disorder. Most have bipolar II disorder (with hypomania). The clinical features of bipolar SAD do not seem different from those of unipolar SAD (Table 1.4), except that hospitalization rates are higher (and primarily due to manic episodes).

Because there may be differences in treatment, it is important to screen for and diagnose bipolar disorder. However, the diagnosis is easy to miss, particularly the less severe hypomanic episodes. The elevated mood and increased energy in the spring is such a relief from the winter depression that many patients do not recognize symptoms or seek help. Often, only close friends and relatives are aware that they are not their usual selves, so obtaining collateral information is very helpful when hypomania is suspected. A summer assessment visit can also help detect people with bipolar disorder.

Clinical example

Sandra looks forward each year to her "summer self", which she sees as ideal: she has much more energy, needs less sleep and is more productive than her depressed "winter self". She sees the summer as a time to make up for the lost winter months, and so throws herself into multiple projects. Her doctor noticed that she seemed to be hypomanic during a routine summer visit, and subsequent collateral information revealed a history of marked irritability that was adversely affecting her relationships and work performance. A diagnosis of "Bipolar II disorder, with seasonal pattern" was made, and treatment adjusted accordingly.

Atypical depression

The reverse neurovegetative features can also be seen in patients with nonseasonal depression with "atypical features" (defined as mood reactivity plus two of the following four symptoms: increased appetite/weight gain, hypersomnia, leaden paralysis, and long-standing interpersonal rejection sensitivity). These patients may happen to be depressed during winter but exploration of their lifetime pattern of depressive episodes will not reveal a seasonal pattern. Conversely, SAD patients are less likely to experience rejection sensitivity and often do not meet full criteria for atypical depression.

Variants of SAD

If people do not have full remissions in summer, they do not technically meet DSM-IV criteria for SAD. However, we and others have noted that many patients with more chronic, year-round depression can experience marked worsening of symptoms in the fall/winter. Several potential variants of winter depression can be postulated (Table 1.6), but seasonal worsening of nonseasonal depression remains an understudied phenomenon.

Subsyndromal SAD

While SAD is considered a categorical diagnosis in DSM-IV (either you have it, or you don't), it can also be conceptualized as a dimensional trait (you can be more or less seasonal) with SAD at the extreme end of the spectrum. The term subsyndromal SAD is often used to describe people who may have many of the signs and symptoms of winter depression, but not to the point where they meet DSM-IV criteria for MDE with seasonal pattern. Subsyndromal SAD can describe several different symptom presentations (Table 1.7). In the DSM-IV, these would be classified as Depressive Disorder, Not Otherwise Specified.

Finally, there are many other people who notice definite changes with winter that are not clinically significant, in that they do not cause personal distress and do not interfere with normal functioning. There is a normal

Table 1.6. Possible variants of winter depression (not in DSM-IV).

Winter episodes	Summer episodes	Possible diagnosis
Major depressive episodes	Full summer remission	Recurrent MDD with seasonal pattern (SAD)
Minor depressive episodes	Full summer remission	Subsyndromal SAD
Major depressive episodes	Residual symptoms	Recurrent MDD without full inter-episode recovery and with seasonal worsening
Major depressive episodes	Minor depressive episodes	Dysthymic disorder with recurrent MDD with seasonal worsening
Major depressive episodes, worse than in summer	Major depressive episodes	Chronic MDD with winter worsening

Table 1.7. Various definitions and presentations for subsyndromal SAD.

- People who do not have the minimum five required symptoms for MDE.
- People who describe a fluctuating course in which symptoms may be significant but never last for the sustained two weeks minimum necessary for MDE.
- People who have significant neurovegetative symptoms (oversleeping, overeating, fatigue) but do not have mood changes or loss of interest.

variation in seasonality within the general population that it is not necessary to label as an illness.

Incomplete summer remission

Clinicians who treat patients with mood disorders recognize that many have winter MDEs but are not in full remission in summer and so do not meet

DSM-IV criteria for seasonal pattern (Table 1.6). Some of these patients have mild depressive symptoms in the summer or only brief periods of remission, suggesting that these are residual depressive symptoms. Others have more symptoms in summer, but not to the point of meeting full criteria for MDE. These patients may have dysthymic disorder, a chronic, low-grade depressive disorder that is punctuated by episodic MDEs (the so-called "double depressions").

Clinical example

Ethan described years of low-grade depressive symptoms over both winter and summer. In the past few years he had clear MDEs during the winter, but in summer he had fewer and milder symptoms. His chronic dysthymic disorder had progressed into a double depression with winter MDEs.

Still others are clearly depressed all year long, with full MDEs during the summer, but worsening substantially in the winter. These patients can be classified as having chronic MDD with winter worsening. Interestingly, some of these patients will experience different depressive symptoms between summer and winter, e.g., they will have melancholic symptoms (insomnia, decreased appetite) when depressed during the summer, but more typical SAD symptoms (oversleeping, overeating) in the winter.

Clinical tip

Studies indicate that people with variants of SAD – minor seasonal depression, SAD with incomplete summer remission, chronic depression with winter worsening – also respond to light treatment. Light treatment may also benefit those with nonseasonal depression. Therefore, the diagnosis of SAD is not necessary to prescribe light treatment.

The importance of these distinctions may not only be semantic. One theory of SAD conceptualizes two interacting processes – one that produces vulnerability to depression and the other vulnerability to seasonality.

Different loadings on these factors may result in these varied presentations for seasonal depression (see Chapter 5). From a clinical perspective, light therapy appears to be effective for these other presentations as well.

Further reading

Blazer DG, Kessler RC, Swartz MS. Epidemiology of recurrent major and minor depression with a seasonal pattern. *Br J Psychiatry* 1998; **172**:164–167.

Lam RW, Tam EM, Yatham LN, Shiah IS, Zis AP. Seasonal depression: the dual vulnerability hypothesis revisited. *J Affect Disord* 2001; **63**:123–132.

Levitt AJ, Boyle MH, Joffe RT, Baumal Z. Estimated prevalence of the seasonal subtype of major depression in a Canadian community sample. *Can J Psychiatry* 2000; **45**:650–654.

Levitt AJ, Boyle MH. The impact of latitude on the prevalence of seasonal depression. *Can J Psychiatry* 2002; **47**:361–367.

Magnusson A, Partonen T. The diagnosis, symptomatology, and epidemiology of seasonal affective disorder. *CNS Spectr* 2005; **10**:625–634.

Mersch PP, Vastenburg NC, Meesters Y, Bouhuys AL, Beersma DG, Van den Hoofdakker RH, den Boer JA. The reliability and validity of the Seasonal Pattern Assessment Questionnaire: a comparison between patient groups. *J Affect Disord* 2004; **80**:209–219.

Michalak EE, Tam EM, Manjunath CV, Enns M, Levitan RD, Morehouse RA, Levitt AJ, Yatham LN, Lam RW. Generic and health-related quality of life in patients with seasonal and nonseasonal depression. *Psychiatry Res* 2004; **128**:245–251.

Partonen T, Magnusson A (eds). *Seasonal Affective Disorder: Practice and Research.* 2nd edition. New York: Oxford University Press, 2009.

Rosenthal NE, Sack DA, Gillin JC, Lewy AJ, Goodwin FK, Davenport Y, Mueller PS, Newsome DA, Wehr TA. Seasonal affective disorder: a description of the syndrome and preliminary findings with light therapy. *Arch Gen Psychiatry* 1984; **41**:72–80.

Schlager D, Froom J, Jaffe A. Winter depression and functional impairment among ambulatory primary care patients. *Compr Psychiatry* 1995; **36**:18–24.

Sohn CH, Lam RW. Treatment of seasonal affective disorder: unipolar versus bipolar differences. *Curr Psychiatr Rep* 2004; **6**:478–485.

Swedo SE, Allen AJ, Glod CA, Clark CH, Teicher MH, Richter D, Hoffman C, Hamburger SD, Dow S, Brown C, Rosenthal NE. A controlled trial of light therapy for the treatment of pediatric seasonal affective disorder. *J Am Acad Child Adolesc Psychiatry* 1997; **36**:816–21.

Westrin Å, Lam RW. Seasonal affective disorder: a clinical update. *Ann Clin Psychiatry* 2007; **19**:239–246.

2

Light Treatment

Incorporate light therapy into clinical practice

Light therapy is easy to "prescribe" and to incorporate into your clinical practice. In this section, we present a step-by-step treatment approach for light therapy based on controlled trials and our own clinical experience. This simplified approach combines proven efficacy with ease of use and improved adherence. In our clinical studies, about two-thirds of patients with SAD will have a robust and satisfactory response to this method. In subsequent sections, we will deconstruct each treatment parameter of light therapy so that individual adjustments can be made, either for patient comfort or because of less than optimal response.

Table 2.1 shows a sample summary visit schedule for a person being evaluated for SAD and treated using a course of light therapy. Further information about the tasks for each visit will be detailed in this chapter.

Encourage self-care

Although light therapy is an effective treatment, people with depression often require a number of interventions to help them recover full functioning. Self-management is an important aspect of care for chronic and recurrent conditions such as depression. People can learn strategies to cope with the symptoms and consequences of depression, and to become active collaborators in the management of their illness.

Education is very important to set the stage for light therapy. Patients need to understand the rationale, benefits and risks, time course of response, and proper methods for light therapy. Providing a variety of educational materials (patient handouts, reading lists, Internet resources) helps to establish a collaborative relationship for treatment and reinforces adherence. Many of the resources that we use in our clinic are provided in Chapter 7 (Clinician Resources), including handouts for Frequently Asked Questions about SAD, self-care tips and patient instructions for light therapy.

Table 2.1. Sample summary visits for assessment of SAD and treatment with light therapy.

	Screening visit	Baseline visit	Follow-up visits	Summer visit
Timing	First visit	Second visit	Every 1–2 weeks until clinical remission is achieved	Summer
Objectives	• Diagnostic assessment • Screen for SAD (if necessary) • Educate about illness	• Initiate light therapy	• Monitor response and side effects • Ensure adherence to treatment • Plan for rest of season (at clinical remission)	• Confirm diagnosis • Plan for next season
Tasks	• Assess diagnosis • Screen for SAD (if necessary) • Assess baseline severity using a rating scale • Send for laboratory tests (if necessary) • Refer for baseline eye testing (if necessary) • Provide patient resources (FAQ, Self-care Tips) • Discuss how to get a light device	• Instruct on use of light device • Provide patient resources (Instructions for Light Therapy) • Assess baseline severity using a rating scale • Discuss potential side effects • Address any treatment adherence issues	• Assess severity and response using a rating scale • Assess side effects • Address any treatment adherence issues • Optimize light therapy parameters • Use other treatments (if necessary) • Discuss continuation treatment for the rest of the season (at clinical remission)	• Assess summer symptoms (depression/hypomania) • Discuss preventative treatment for next season • Address any treatment adherence issues
Comments	• Depending on the setting, the screening and baseline visits may be combined. • In primary care settings, people may not be aware that they have a depressive disorder or SAD when coming for this visit. Therefore, the groundwork needs to be done prior to active treatment, i.e., making sure the person understands the illness and potential treatments. • In mental health settings, people may be referred specifically for light therapy, and so will be ready to initiate treatment when the diagnostic assessment is complete.		• Number and frequency of follow-up visits will depend on severity of symptoms and response to treatment. • People with higher severity of symptoms may need to be seen once a week, especially in the early phase of treatment. • The summer assessment is very informative for diagnostic issues, especially to detect bipolar II disorder.	

Who should not use light therapy?

There are no absolute contraindications to light therapy and it is a safe procedure when used according to these guidelines (see "Bright light toxicity"). However, bright light may be relatively contraindicated in some patients because of the potential to aggravate underlying retinal conditions. These include people with pre-existing retinal diseases and systemic diseases that can affect the eye, and those taking photosensitizing medications. People with these risk factors who are considering light therapy should have a baseline ophthalmological assessment and then regular follow-up assessments at least annually.

> **Clinical tip**
>
> Remember to let people know that tanning salons are NOT effective for SAD. The antidepressant effects of light are mediated through the eyes, not the skin. Recommended light devices filter out the ultraviolet wavelengths so as not to damage the eyes.

Use the simplified light treatment method

This method is based on the use of the "gold standard" light device: a fluorescent light box designed to produce 10,000 lux white light at a specified distance from the eyes of the user (Table 2.2). There is an approximate relationship between intensity and duration of exposure, so that people using light devices with lower lux ratings usually need longer daily exposure time. For example, 5,000 lux light boxes require 45 minutes to 1 hour of daily exposure, while 2,500 lux light boxes require at least 2 hours. Other light devices may have different treatment parameters (see Chapter 3).

Lux is a measure of illumination intensity adjusted to the wavelengths visible to the human eye. It can be described as the brightness of light reflected from a surface. The lux rating varies by several orders of magnitude in our daily environment. For example:

Indoor lighting:
- Living room with floor lamps – 100 lux
- Fluorescent-lit office – 300 lux
- The brightest possible room light – 500 lux

Outdoor light:
- Gray, cloudy winter day – 3,000 lux
- Snowy overcast winter day – 5,000 lux
- Sunny midday – 50,000 to 100,000 lux or higher

A rating of 10,000 lux is equivalent to being outdoors, looking away from the sun, about an hour after sunrise on the summer solstice (June 21).

Table 2.2.	Summary of recommendations for light therapy.

1. Gold standard device: fluorescent light box that emits 10,000 lux white light, with a filter to screen out ultraviolet wavelengths.
2. Start with 30 minutes in the early morning upon waking (preferably before 9:00 a.m., ideally 7:00 a.m. or earlier).
3. If not using a 10,000 lux light box, follow manufacturer's recommendation for exposure duration.
4. Use light therapy daily for the duration of the fall/winter season until past the usual offset time of the winter depressive episode.
5. Customize the parameters of treatment to suit the individual patient.

The light box is usually used at home (although in Europe there are "light rooms" in hospital clinics, and "light cafes" with light boxes at each table so that bright light can be experienced while having one's morning coffee or breakfast). The user sits in front of the 10,000 lux light box for 30 minutes each day, starting as soon as possible in the early morning upon awakening (usually between 7:00 a.m. and 9:00 a.m.). Users should not stare directly at the light. Instead, they can be reading or eating breakfast, as long as their eyes are open to receive the light. After using the light, people can resume their usual daily activities.

Response to light therapy is usually quite rapid. There is an immediate energizing effect of bright light which helps to keep people awake and eases the sleep inertia that is experienced by most patients with SAD. The antidepressant effect of light (i.e., specific effects on other symptoms of depression) may take a bit longer, but many people notice improvement of symptoms starting within 1 week. For others, the response may be somewhat slower, so that 2 or 3 weeks may be needed before they experience significant improvement. However, if absolutely no response is seen by 2 weeks, we recommend changing a treatment parameter (see "Trouble-shoot poor or limited response").

> **Clinical tip**
>
> Some people experience the energizing effect of light as uncomfortable, like a feeling of being tense, on edge, or speedy. If this happens, it usually resolves with reducing the light exposure by sitting a little farther away from the light box or spending less time under the lights.

Some studies have examined predictors of response to light therapy. Patients with atypical vegetative symptoms (oversleeping, overeating, carbohydrate craving) tend to have higher response rates to bright light. However, the predictive value of atypical features is not particularly helpful because the response rate is still good for people with other symptoms.

Monitor clinical response

It is very important for patients and clinicians to monitor clinical response during light treatment. Clinical guidelines for treatment of MDD recommend that patients be treated to full remission because the presence of residual depressive symptoms is associated with poorer long-term outcomes. Without proper monitoring, it is difficult to determine whether and when patients achieve full remission.

Most clinicians use only a global impression of response to guide treatment decisions. This usually involves asking the patient how they are doing and whether they notice a difference since starting treatment. While global impressions can be useful, they can also be misleading and lead to incorrect treatment decisions (see "Clinical scenarios" below). Only by checking each individual symptom is it possible to determine the degree of response. For this reason, we recommend using a symptom rating scale to monitor the patient's response. Using rating scales, we can define clinical response as 50% reduction in the total score – noticeable improvement by both patient and clinician. Clinical remission is usually defined as a score in the normal or not depressed range. Non-response is often defined as 20% or less reduction in total score.

Clinical scenario 1

After 2 weeks of light therapy, Sandra returns and says, "I'm not feeling any better – the lights must not be working". The global impression indicates that the dose of light should be increased. However, when each symptom is examined, there is slight improvement in many symptoms, and these add up to indicate mild but definite overall improvement. Consequently, Sandra was advised to not change her treatment parameters and to wait for a couple more weeks to gauge response.

Clinical scenario 2

After 4 weeks of light therapy, Sandra returns and says "I'm feeling a lot better – the lights must be working". The global impression indicates no change in treatment is needed. However, on closer questioning, she still has many residual symptoms and is not in clinical remission. She was therefore advised to increase the dose of light to see whether further improvement could be obtained.

In both these scenarios, the initial global impression was misleading and the correct treatment advice was indicated only after checking all the symptoms.

Rating scales can be administered by a clinical interview or can be self-rated by patients. The most widely used clinician-rated depression scale is the Hamilton Depression Rating Scale (Ham-D). The Ham-D has been adapted for use in SAD and a structured interview guide (the SIGH-SAD) has been used in many studies. The SIGH-SAD takes about 20 minutes to complete.

There is good correlation between patient-rated and clinician-rated scales and, for busy practices, patient self-rated scales are usually more efficient than a full clinical interview. Patients can complete and score a rating scale at home prior to the clinic appointment, or in the waiting room upon arrival. The clinician can then review the scale results with the patient during the visit. Commonly used self-rating scales include the Patient Health Questionnaire (PHQ-9) and the Quick Inventory of Depressive Symptomatology, Self-Rated (QIDS-SR). Both of these scales are based on the nine symptom criteria for MDD. The PHQ-9 is useful in a primary care setting because it can also be used to aid diagnosis as well as monitor treatment. The QIDS-SR is slightly better at measuring severity of symptoms and was used in the STAR*D effectiveness study. Some examples of clinician- and patient-rated scales are included in Chapter 7 (Clinician Resources).

Manage side effects

Most people tolerate light therapy quite well and rarely does anyone drop out of a treatment trial due to side effects. Table 2.3 summarizes several clinical studies on side effects of light therapy. The self-rated Adverse Events Scale used in the CAN-SAD study is included in Chapter 7 (Clinician Resources), but it is probably more detailed than necessary for clinical practice. Nonetheless, it can be useful to track and monitor side effects in some patients, such as those who are particularly sensitive to side effects of treatment.

At our clinic, the most common nuisance side effects that patients spontaneously report are eye dryness or irritation, headache, and feeling "wired". These adverse effects usually can be eased by sitting slightly farther away from the light box (thereby reducing the intensity of light) or slightly reducing the treatment time. Often side effects subside with time, which then allows the patient to readjust the treatment "dose" upwards again.

Table 2.3.	Reported adverse effects of light therapy (10,000 lux fluorescent light box, 30 minutes/day) for SAD in three studies. Only side effects reported in more than 5% of treated patients are shown.

Study	Kogan and Guilford, 1998	Terman and Terman, 1999	Lam et al., 2006.[a]
Length of treatment and sample size:	4 to 10 days, n=70	10 to 14 days, n=83	8 weeks, n=48
Emergent side effect	%	%	%
Gastrointestinal			
Abdominal discomfort/pain		10	6
Nausea/vomiting	7	16	4
Diarrhea		13	4
Constipation		2	8
Appetite/weight			
Decreased appetite		19	15
Increased appetite		15	8
Weight loss		19	2
Weight gain		10	
Central nervous system			
Headache	21	8	17
Fatigue/weakness	6	3	8–17
Increased sleep		9	13
Decreased sleep		7–14	23
Overactive/excited/ agitated	6	9–10	
Anxiety	3	5	13

Table 2.3.   (cont.)

Sexual dysfunction			
Decreased sexual interest			
Increased sexual interest		18	
Difficulties with orgasm		6	
Difficulties with erection		5	5
Eyes/Ear/Nose/Throat			
Eye or vision problem	19	4–6	
Mouth sores		8	
Nasal congestion		12	
Dry mouth/throat		4–8	19
Chest			
Shortness of breath		6	
Coughing		15	
Breast tenderness		6	
Other			
Muscle/bone/joint pain		8	13
Fever/chills		7	
Sweating/flushing			6
Feeling faint			6

[a] Unlike most clinical trials that depend on spontaneous patient reports, these studies used systematic questionnaires to detect treatment-emergent adverse events.

Clinical example

Ethan initially found light therapy irritating because of a headache that persisted for a few hours after treatment. The headaches improved when he reduced his treatment time to 20 minutes a day. After a few days the headaches went away and he was then able to continue light therapy for 30 minutes.

Serious side effects

Like other effective antidepressant treatments, light therapy potentially can cause a switch to a hypomanic or manic state. Although such a switch is relatively rare, it is important for patients and clinicians to be aware of this serious side effect. Patients with bipolar disorder or vulnerability to bipolar disorder (e.g., a positive family history) are at higher risk. We recommend that patients with Bipolar I disorder be on a mood stabilizing medication when using light therapy.

Clinical example

Sandra reported a history of hypomanic symptoms (agitation, racing thoughts, hyperactivity) when traveling to sunny southern places in the summer. With light therapy she experienced side effects very similar to these symptoms and so she reduced the treatment time to 15 minutes a day. Her side effects resolved and she still found benefit with the shorter treatment duration.

A couple of case reports suggested that some patients using light treatment may experience increasing suicidal thoughts as a side effect. Suicidality (worsening suicidal ideas and behaviours) has been a controversial concern with antidepressant medications and some wondered whether it might also apply to light therapy. Closer examination in larger SAD samples found no evidence that light therapy was associated with increased suicidality. In fact, treatment with light therapy resulted in significant reduction in suicidal ideas.

Clinical tip

It is always important to monitor depressed patients carefully in the first few weeks when starting any treatment, whether light therapy, pharmacotherapy, or psychotherapy. This is a high-risk period for suicidal ideas because patients are usually feeling worse when first presenting for treatment and because the treatments have not yet begun to help.

Bright light toxicity

Very bright light exposure has been shown to have toxic effects on the retina in animal studies, so there has been attention to the retinal safety of bright light therapy. Several studies of long-term use of light therapy have not shown any adverse effects on the retina. Given that the light produced is only about as bright as summer morning light and that the ultraviolet wavelengths are filtered out, any potential for retinal toxicity is minimal.

Nonetheless, some individuals may be at higher risk for eye toxicity to bright light (Table 2.4). Some patients have pre-existing retinal disease such as retinitis pigmentosa while others have a medical illness, such as diabetes, which can involve the retina. Still others may be on photosensitizing medications such as lithium, phenothiazine antipsychotics, melatonin and St. John's wort (hypericum). All patients should be screened for these risk factors on initial assessment. For these patients, we recommend an ophthalmological examination prior to treatment, and regular checks at least annually.

Clinical tip

Routine eye examinations are not necessary for most people starting light therapy. However, we recommend baseline and regular follow-up examinations for those with risk factors for potential bright light toxicity.

The human retina is particularly sensitive to blue light and there is a well-described "blue light hazard" consisting of retinal damage with exposure to high-intensity blue light sources (such as welding torches). It is unlikely that the blue light hazard will be a problem with lower-intensity blue light. However, because of the potential for toxicity and without any long-term safety data, we do not recommend blue light devices for light therapy.

Table 2.4. Risk factors for potential toxicity with bright light exposure.

Pre-existing retinal or eye disease:
- retinal detachment
- retinitis pigmentosa
- macular degeneration
- glaucoma

Systemic illnesses that affect the retina
- diabetes mellitus
- rheumatoid arthritis
- systemic lupus erythematosus

Photosensitizing medications:
- lithium
- phenothiazines, such as thioridazine (antipsychotics, antiemetics)
- melatonin
- St. John's wort (hypericum)
- chloroquine (used to treat malaria)
- hematoporphyrins (used in cancer treatment)
- 8-methoxypsoralens (used in psoriasis treatment)

Older age:
- may have undetected age-related macular degeneration

Enhance adherence

Using light therapy daily requires motivation and commitment of time. Follow-up studies of people with SAD show that many stop using their lights, even if they received substantial benefit from treatment. This is not surprising because we know how challenging it is for people to incorporate healthy behaviours into their daily routine, whether these are exercise, stress reduction, taking a medication or using light treatment. Therefore, encouraging treatment adherence should be a routine activity at every visit.

One major barrier to adherence is that patients with hypersomnia find it very difficult to wake up early enough to use the lights. Once response begins, usually within a week or two, it gets easier to wake up on time. Until then, patients may find these tips helpful for their morning schedule:

- Use two alarms. Most people like to set their clock radio to awaken to music, but a second annoying buzzer set 5 or 10 minutes later is often more effective.
- Use wake-up telephone calls. There are inexpensive telephone services available which will ring you up at a pre-set wake time, with frequent reminder calls. Or, enlist a friend or relative to help out by calling for the first week of treatment.
- Set the bedroom lights to a timer. It is much easier to awaken into light than into darkness, and the extra step of turning on a light often makes it easier to fall back asleep. Although not true "dawn simulation" (see Chapter 3), setting the lights to come on with your alarm can be very helpful.
- Keep the light box or device in the bedroom to use as soon as possible upon waking.

Patients also can be tempted to skip the light therapy when feeling better. One strategy to encourage regular use of light is to chart treatment use between appointments. Keeping a journal of light therapy times helps to maintain the schedule until it becomes a habit. The clinician can help by reviewing this "homework" at follow-up visits. If patients chart their moods at the same time, the journal also can be used to help track clinical response.

Customize treatment

Once people have a response to light therapy, it may be helpful to customize the parameters of treatment to make it more convenient to use and to enhance long-term adherence. Since light therapy works quite quickly, one can change a treatment parameter and wait a week or two to monitor changes in mood and other symptoms to evaluate the effects of the change. If worsening occurs, then patients can revert to the previous setting. Remember that it is easier to monitor response to parameter changes if a symptom rating scale is used!

For example, some people may be able to maintain their response with shorter daily exposure time. Reducing exposure to 15–20 minutes per day can be tried for a week or two. If worsening occurs, they can revert to 30 minutes daily.

Similarly, it is usually possible to use light treatment only on weekdays. Missing two days on the weekend is usually not associated with relapse of symptoms (relapse typically takes more than a few days to occur) and it allows people to "take a break" or sleep in on the weekends. Of course, sleeping in too late during the weekends can make it even more difficult to awaken for light treatment on Monday morning. For others, skipping even a couple of days makes it more difficult to keep up a routine, and they prefer to use the light treatment every day.

Clinical tip

Some people also use their light boxes for a brief time (15 minutes or so) in the afternoon to treat the "afternoon slump" in mood and energy.

Some patients may not need morning timing of light. They can try to change the time of light to afternoon or evening, if it is more convenient, to see whether they achieve the same response. If they use evening light exposure, they should not schedule the light in the later evening (past 8:00 p.m. or so) as it might interfere with initiation of sleep.

Clinical tip

Adapting light therapy to the patient's own circumstances is important for adherence: a "sub-optimal" but workable schedule may produce better results than an "optimal" but unworkable schedule.

Review treatment parameters

The simplified method specifies standard "dosing" for light treatment which is beneficial for the majority of patients with SAD. However, there are several treatment parameters that can be adjusted if patients show no response or insufficient response. In this section, we will review the studies of these parameters.

Light intensity (brightness)

How bright does the light have to be, to be effective? To answer this important question requires some consideration about the way that light is measured. Light is a very complex physical phenomenon and there are many ways to measure the intensity of light. For example, we can measure the radiance (the energy produced from photon transfer) or the luminance (the power of visible light matched to the responsivity of the human eye). Historically, lux – a measure of illuminance – has been used to measure intensity of light therapy. However, there is no clear relationship between lux and perceived "brightness" of light. That is because the human retina adapts readily to changes in illumination and the perceived brightness does not indicate how much light actually reaches the retina. For example, it takes a few minutes after entering a dimly lit room before you are able to see clearly. The lux level has not changed during that time; instead, the photoreceptors in your retina have adapted to the low light level.

The lux rating varies with the inverse square of the distance to the light source. That means that when you move twice the distance from the light source, the lux rating drops by four times. Thus, a 10,000 lux rating at 18 inches from a light box becomes only 2,500 lux at 3 feet. You can see that sitting just a little farther away from a light box causes the lux rating to fall dramatically. Similarly, moving a few feet from a window means that you are exposed to typical indoor lux ratings, even on a sunny day. The minimal intensity to demonstrate an antidepressant effect of light is approximately 1,500 lux. The brightest indoor light levels only approach 500 lux, an intensity that has been used as a "placebo condition" in light therapy studies (see Chapter 5).

> **Clinical tip**
>
> The antidepressant effect of light requires an intensity that is at least three times as bright as the brightest indoor light. Therefore, you cannot treat SAD by simply increasing the room light or moving to an office with a window. The 10,000 lux fluorescent light boxes are rated at 20 times as bright as the brightest indoor room light.

Duration of treatment session

The original lower-intensity light boxes studied for light therapy were rated at 2,500 lux and required at least 2 hours of daily exposure. However, 4 hours of light exposure was no better than 2 hours. Studies also showed that 10,000 lux light boxes needed only 30 minutes of daily exposure to show comparable results while 5,000 lux light boxes generally required 45–60 minutes. In contrast, 2,500 lux for 30 minutes did not have much effect. This shows some relationship between the lux intensity and the length of time of exposure, so the "dose" of light therapy can be increased by either increasing the intensity or by increasing the amount of exposure time.

Time of day of treatment

The timing of light treatment has many theoretical implications for the mechanism of action of light (see Chapter 5). In summary, however, the evidence shows that morning light has the greatest therapeutic effect. However, light given at other times of the day may also provide some benefit. Our clinical experience backs the studies showing that some patients are preferential morning responders, hence our recommendation to start with morning light therapy to optimize response. We have not seen many patients who preferentially respond at other times of the day. However, this is not the same as saying that light has no response when given at other times. For some patients, it does not seem to matter what time they receive light. It is possible for them to use the light at a more convenient time of the day.

Wavelength of light

White light is composed of many different wavelengths and has been the most-studied and best-evaluated treatment. The type of light does not seem to matter, so that fluorescent or incandescent or light-emitting diodes all seem to be effective. Similarly, "full spectrum" fluorescent bulbs, which have wavelengths more closely matched to that of sunlight, are no better than other types of fluorescent light, such as cool-white. Halogen lights are not recommended because at the required intensity they tend to be much hotter than other lights. Studies of narrow-wavelength light (which appears as different colours) have many methodological limitations that make them difficult to interpret. However, no specific wavelength or colour of light has ever been shown to be superior to white light.

Recently, there has been attention to blue light, with some claims that it is more effective in treating SAD. In part this was due to significant breakthroughs in our understanding of the effects of light on the biological clock (see Chapter 5). A neural tract connecting the retina to the suprachiasmatic nucleus (the biological pacemaker in the brain) has been known for years, but it was unclear which photoreceptors in the retina were necessary for transducing the light signal. Experiments in animals showed that rod and cone photoreceptors, which are important for vision, were not necessary for light to affect circadian rhythms. Instead, a recent discovery found that melanopsin, a novel photopigment found in retinal glial cells, is the main photoreceptor responsible for circadian effects of light. Characterization of melanopsin has shown that it responds maximally to wavelengths in the blue-green part of the spectrum. Human studies have confirmed that blue light is more efficient in shifting the circadian system, that is, that less intensity is required using blue light than using light of other wavelengths.

Although blue light may have greater efficiency in shifting circadian rhythms, there is still no evidence that it is better for treating SAD or other depressive conditions. One small study has shown that blue light (of low lux intensity) is better than a placebo low-light condition, but another study found that white light was as good as, or slightly better than, the blue light. Because of the potential risk of retinal toxicity with long-term blue light exposure (see "Bright light toxicity"), and because blue light is not superior to white light, we do not recommend blue light devices for light therapy.

Trouble-shoot poor or limited response

If the patient experiences a poor response to light therapy, you should review the method with them and adjust the dosing parameters. We go through the following questions, in roughly this order, and adjust the light therapy method accordingly.

(1) How often are they using the lights?

If patients are not responding as expected, the first thing we check is whether they are actually using the lights. Despite best intentions, patients can sometimes miss days of treatment and not mention this during follow-up. We find it useful to always ask about adherence and to ensure that they are using the lights daily.

(2) Are they using the lights properly?

The next step is to check whether they are properly following the instructions. This includes sitting the correct distance from the light box to receive the proper intensity and making sure that nothing blocks the light from reaching the eyes. Some patients have even worn sunglasses during treatment and wondered why the light therapy was not working!

Clinical tip

The smaller the light device, the smaller is the field of exposure. For very small screens, one needs to be extremely careful about positioning, because even small movements of the head or body may reduce the light intensity.

Clinical example

During a follow-up visit, Ethan reported no benefit of light therapy. However, he had placed the light box atop his refrigerator so as to better illuminate the whole kitchen, not realizing that this reduced the intensity to non-therapeutic levels. Using the light box properly led to a good response.

(3) How long are they using the lights?

The first strategy for poor or partial response to 10,000 lux is to increase the dose of light by increasing the time of exposure. Since most people start with 30 minutes, this can be increased to 45 or 60 minutes daily.

Clinical tip

In our experience, only the most motivated people will be able to spend more than an hour a day using the lights, especially in the long term. People using lower-intensity light boxes who require more than an hour of daily exposure should switch to 10,000 lux. If people do not respond to 10,000 lux at 60 minutes per day, we usually use another strategy rather than recommending a longer exposure time.

(4) What time are they using the lights?

Some people do not use light therapy at an early enough time. They may respond to moving the timing of light to as early as possible. Others may find it more helpful to try light therapy at other times of the day, such as in the afternoon or evening.

Clinical examples

Sandra adamantly reports that she uses the light box "every morning, as soon as she gets up". However, her wake-up time varies greatly, from 7:00 a.m. to 9:30 a.m. She had a better response when she started using the light consistently at 7:00 a.m.

Roger finds it impossible to use the light in the morning, as his schedule is just too busy at that time. Nonetheless, he was determined to try light therapy instead of medications. He decided to try light therapy in the evening, with significant response.

| Table 2.5. | Timing of light therapy based on Morningness-Eveningness Questionnaire Score. Adapted from Terman and Terman, 2005. |

MEQ score	Time to start light therapy
16–18	8:45 a.m.
19–22	8:30 a.m.
23–26	8:15 a.m.
27–30	8:00 a.m.
31–34	7:45 a.m.
35–38	7:30 a.m.
39–41	7:15 a.m.
42–45	7:00 a.m.
46–49	6:45 a.m.
50–53	6:30 a.m.
54–57	6:15 a.m.
58–61	6:00 a.m.
62–65	5:45 a.m.
66–68	5:30 a.m.
69–72	5:15 a.m.
73–76	5:00 a.m.
77–80	4:45 a.m.
81–84	4:30 a.m.
85–86	4:15 a.m.

Alternatively, Dr. Michael Terman has data suggesting that there is an optimal timing for morning light exposure based on the patient's individual circadian rhythm. His study indicated that light therapy should begin about 8.5 hours after the onset of melatonin secretion at night. While it is still difficult to clinically measure melatonin onset, this can be estimated by a score from the self-rated Morningness-Eveningness Questionnaire (MEQ, included in Chapter 7). The MEQ was originally developed to assess chronotype, or whether the person is a morning person (a "lark") or a night person (an "owl"). Interestingly, the MEQ score has also been correlated to circadian measurements such as core body temperature.

Table 2.5 shows the optimal timing of light therapy based on the patient's MEQ score. Although the effectiveness of routine use of this timing schedule has not yet been confirmed, we find it helpful to try it when a patient does not respond to the simplified light treatment method. An on-line automated version of the MEQ with recommended start times for light therapy is available at www.cet.org.

Clinical tip

Remember to try to adjust one parameter at a time, otherwise it will be unclear what has actually worked or not. Since the response to light is rapid, the patient should experience the results of a parameter change within a week or two.

How long to continue light therapy

By definition, SAD is a recurrent depressive condition, so long-term and preventative treatment is indicated. Unfortunately, there is little information on how long light therapy needs to be continued after an initial response, and on preventative use of light treatment in subsequent winter episodes. Some people seem to only need a brief time using light therapy and then are well through the rest of the winter. However, the majority of people who respond to light will usually show relapse of symptoms when the light therapy is stopped. Therefore, most people should use light therapy daily throughout the winter season until the time of their usual spring remission (Table 2.6).

Clinical tip

There are no discontinuation symptoms reported with stopping bright light treatment, so there is no need to taper light exposure.

Table 2.6.	Recommendations for continuation and preventative treatment.

Continuation treatment
- Patients should continue to use daily light therapy until the time of their usual spring/summer remission (i.e., usually by end of April)
- Some patients may find it useful to use light treatment in the summer (e.g., during extended bouts of cloudy weather)

Preventative treatment
- To prevent an episode, most patients should re-start light treatment in the fall, about 2 weeks prior to the usual onset of symptoms (e.g., if symptoms start in November, begin using lights in mid-October)
- Some patients may wish to wait until first onset of symptoms before starting light therapy. If so, completing mood rating scales weekly around the time of usual symptom onset helps to identify early symptoms

When to restart light treatment in a subsequent season

There are no good studies on the best strategy for preventing episodes of winter depression after a season of treatment. The choice of when to start treatment with light depends on the individual. Because of the rapidity of effect of light therapy, some people can wait for first symptoms before starting treatment. Others prefer to start treatment well before onset of symptoms in the early fall, to fully avert an episode. Table 2.7 shows some of the questions to consider for this decision.

Using light therapy in the summer

Some people with SAD find that their mood dips in the summer, especially during extended periods of cloudy or rainy weather. The use of light therapy during these times can be helpful to optimize mood and function in the summer. Again, they should be cautioned about the overuse of light as it might produce more agitation or mild hypomanic symptoms in the summer.

Table 2.7.   Questions to consider in the decision about preventative treatment and when to start light therapy.

- How many past episodes have there been?
- How regular is the pattern of episodes, i.e., do episodes occur every year, or will they skip some years?
- How regular and predictable is the time of onset of symptoms?
- How slowly do symptoms come on?
- How quickly do they respond to light?

Clinical examples

Roger has regular episodes every year starting in mid-November and his symptoms progress rapidly to impairment. He starts light therapy before onset of symptoms, in late October. That way, he prevents an episode entirely.

Vicky has had five previous episodes of winter depression but noticed a couple of past years when she "skipped" a season and did not have many winter symptoms. Her episode onset is also somewhat variable, with symptoms starting in October some years, and later in November in others. She has slow progression of symptoms, so that she notices increased need for sleep, low energy and fatigue some weeks before other depressive symptoms impair her function. She likes to wait until onset of these physical symptoms before she starts using her light box.

Sandra has regular winter episodes with variable onset between October and December. While her symptoms are slow to progress, in past years she has waited too long before starting light therapy. Before she realized it, she was in a full-blown episode of depression and then lacked motivation and energy to start using lights again. Now she rates her depressive symptoms once a week in the autumn using the PHQ-9. When her score begins to rise, she knows she should start using her lights again.

Clinical tip

A scheduled summer follow-up visit can be very helpful to (1) check for summer remission, (2) check for hypomania (perhaps indicating a bipolar II disorder), (3) advise about summer treatment, and (4) discuss preventative treatment for the upcoming winter season.

Further reading

Baehr EK, Revelle W, Eastman CI. Individual differences in the phase and amplitude of the human circadian temperature rhythm: with an emphasis on morningness-eveningness. *J Sleep Res* 2000; **9**:117–127.

Gallin PF, Terman M, Reme CE, Rafferty B, Terman JS, Burde RM. Ophthalmologic examination of patients with seasonal affective disorder, before and after bright light therapy. *Am J Ophthalmol* 1995; **119**:202–210.

Kogan AO, Guilford PM. Side effects of short-term 10,000-lux light therapy. *Am J Psychiatry* 1998; **155**:293–294.

Lam RW, Levitt AJ (eds). *Canadian Consensus Guidelines for the Treatment of Seasonal Affective Disorder*. Vancouver, BC: Clinical and Academic Publishing, 1999.

Reme CE, Rol P, Grothmann K, Kaase H, Terman M. Bright light therapy in focus: lamp emission spectra and ocular safety. *Technol Health Care* 1996; **4**:403–413.

Terman JS, Terman M, Lo ES, Cooper TB. Circadian time of morning light administration and therapeutic response in winter depression. *Arch Gen Psychiatry* 2001; **58**:69–75.

Terman M, Terman JS. Bright light therapy: side effects and benefits across the symptom spectrum. *J Clin Psychiatry* 1999; **60**:799–808.

Terman M, Terman JS. Light therapy for seasonal and nonseasonal depression: efficacy, protocol, safety, and side effects. *CNS Spectr* 2005; **10**:647–663.

Westrin Å, Lam RW. Long-term and preventative treatment for seasonal affective disorder. *CNS Drugs* 2007; **21**:901–909.

Light Devices

What to look for in a light device

The good news is that light devices for treating SAD and other conditions are now widely available. They are now stocked in many retail outlets, including department stores (e.g., Sears), drugstores or pharmacies, and medical supply shops. They are also available for purchase over the Internet.

The bad news, however, is that devices for light therapy are still an unregulated industry and there are no accepted standards for these devices. And, there are many unsubstantiated claims being made by companies. While light boxes have been the "gold standard" device, newer devices have also been tested and found effective. However, there are many types of devices being sold that have never been evaluated or proven effective for the treatment of SAD. The situation is still best described as "buyer beware".

Since we still do not know exactly how light therapy works, and given the many types of devices and claims, it is prudent to be cautious about recommending a specific device. We believe it is important to consider the following questions when purchasing a light device:

1) What is the evidence for that type of device being effective?
2) Has that particular device been used in scientifically valid clinical studies?
3) Has the device been safety-tested by an approved agency (e.g., CSA in Canada or UL in the United States)?
4) Does the device have a filter to block ultraviolet wavelengths (which are not necessary for the antidepressant response, and which are potentially harmful with long-term exposure)?
5) What is the warranty and return policy for the device?
6) What is the track record of reliability for the device company, e.g., how long has it been in business?

Note that we do NOT recommend that people build their own light devices, because of the potential electrical hazards and the difficulty in achieving the required intensity of light. As previously mentioned, we also recommend white light devices, as there is no indication that blue light is more effective, there are theoretical reasons for blue light toxicity, and the safety of blue light devices has not yet been adequately evaluated in clinical studies.

> **Clinical tip**
>
> The Circadian Lighting Association (CLA) is an international group of device manufacturers that has agreed to abide by a Code of Practice to ensure that consumers have appropriate knowledge to guide purchase decisions. The CLA web site (www.claorg.org) has useful information about light devices and how to obtain them.

Light boxes

The fluorescent light box is the most widely used and studied light device, and so it remains the standard recommendation for light therapy. The original light boxes were enormous: eight four-foot fluorescent tubes mounted in a large box with reflective material that was rated at 2,500 lux, requiring 2–4 hours of exposure per day. Now, the 10,000 lux light boxes are more compact and easier to use, requiring only 30 minutes of daily exposure. Fluorescent bulbs are safe, energy-efficient and long-lasting. There is no indication that the more expensive full-spectrum fluorescent bulbs are any better for light therapy than cool-white or others. For reasons described in Chapter 2, we do not recommend halogen or blue-light devices.

Some important aspects when comparing light boxes include glare and size of screen. Many light boxes are mounted on a stand so that the light is fixed above and at an angle to the user (Figure 3.1). This allows the light to reach the eyes but reduces the glare from direct exposure to the light source so that users can read comfortably. A diffusing screen also helps to reduce glare. Some of the smaller light devices have a limited screen size for the light source. This means that positioning of the device is very important, as even small changes in posture or positioning will reduce the lux rating. Devices with larger screens have less variability of lux rating with positioning.

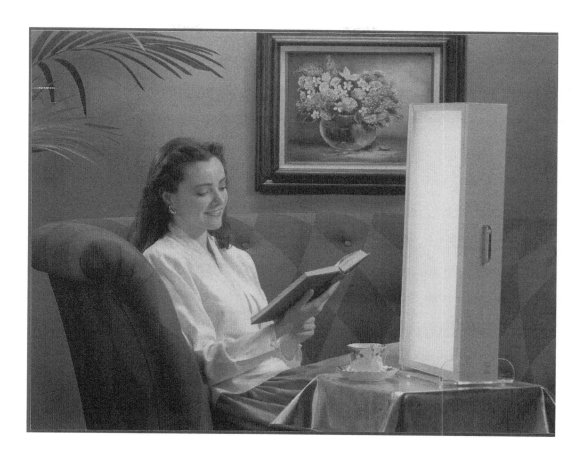

Figure 3.1a Examples of fluorescent light boxes from reputable companies. (a) Photo courtesy of Enviro-Med, www.bio-light.com. (b) Photo courtesy of Uplift Technologies Inc., www.day-lights.com. (c) Photo courtesy of Northern Light Technologies, www. northernlighttechnologies.com. (d) Photo from Philips, www.lighttherapy.com.

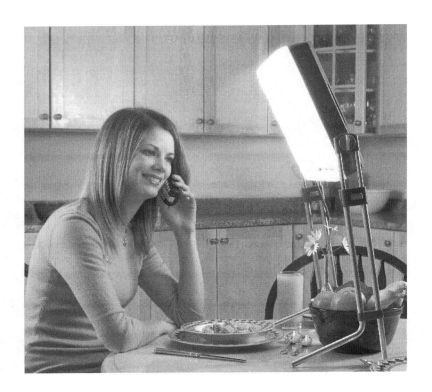

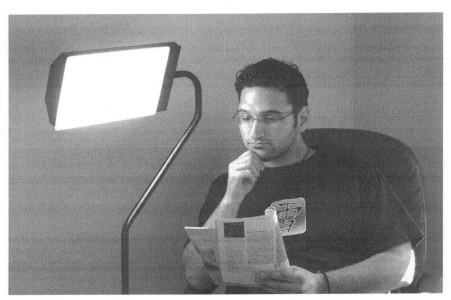

Figure 3.1b, c

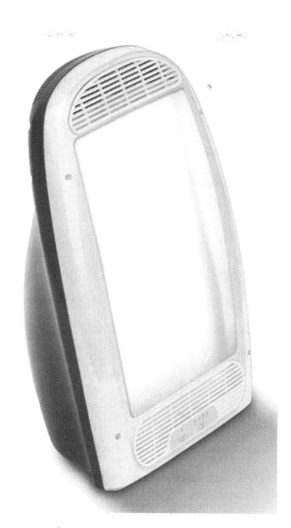

Figure 3.1d

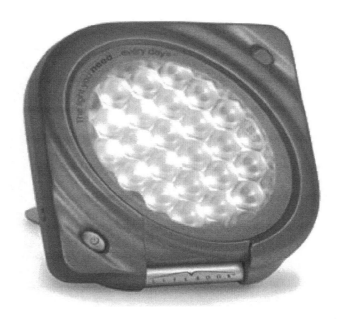

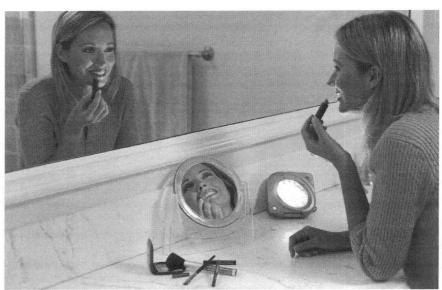

Figure 3.2.   An example of an LED device. Photo courtesy of Litebook, www.litebook.com.

LED devices

Recently, there has been interest in light devices using light-emitting diodes (LEDs). An advantage of LEDs is that they can achieve high intensity brightness in a smaller surface area, so the devices are smaller and more portable than most light boxes (Figure 3.2). They also require less power and can be run on batteries, thereby obviating the need for an electrical cord and outlet. LEDs are energy-efficient and last forever (or almost forever) so they never need replacement.

Preliminary clinical studies have shown that white-light LED devices are also effective in treating SAD (Figure 3.3). Of interest is that the lux rating for LED devices is much lower than the 10,000 lux light boxes, but the response rates appear similar even though the exposure time in LED studies was limited to 30 minutes. It is possible that there are other differences in the light wavelengths of LED devices that make them more efficient than fluorescent light boxes.

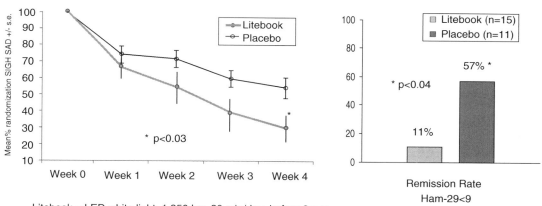

Litebook = LED white light, 1,350 lux, 30 min/day, before 8 a.m.
Placebo = Inactive negative ion generator

Figure 3.3 Results from a placebo-controlled RCT of an LED light device for SAD. Figure adapted from: Desan PH, Weinstein AJ, Michalak EE, Tam EM, Meesters Y, Ruiter MJ, Horn E, Telner J, Iskandar H, Boivin DB, Lam RW. A controlled trial of the Litebook light-emitting diode (LED) light therapy device for treatment of Seasonal Affective Disorder (SAD). *BMC Psychiatry* 2007; 7:38.

The small size of these devices is also a potential disadvantage because of the narrow illumination angles, making the lux intensity particularly vulnerable to changes in positioning. Users need to make sure that they are positioned and using the LED device properly to achieve the rated lux intensity.

If size or portability is an important consideration, then one can choose the smaller LED devices. People with limited desk space in their home or office, or who travel often, will find the LED device less cumbersome than a light box. However, more studies will need to be done before they can be recommended with the same degree of confidence as fluorescent light boxes.

Light visors and caps

Another attempt to improve portability involved light visors or light caps. These devices had small battery-operated lights (usually incandescent) mounted on the visor and positioned to shine into the eyes. Theoretically, users could then move around and continue their daily activities while receiving light therapy.

Prior to 1995, three studies were conducted using similar light visors. All were very well designed and had large sample sizes. However, in contrast to the results of many fluorescent light box studies, all three visor studies were unable to demonstrate the effectiveness of the bright light condition against a dim light placebo condition. The light visors did not seem to show the same clinical effects as light boxes, although the reasons for this are still unclear. Given the uncertainty of these clinical effects, light visors are not recommended as a first-choice light device.

Dawn simulators

Another variation on light therapy is based on the theory that the dawn signal is most important in correcting circadian rhythm disturbances and that people with SAD need a "summer dawn" which starts much earlier than a winter dawn. This is done with a dawn simulator – a device that mimics a

summer dawn in the bedroom. The dawn simulator is essentially
a programmable timer that controls a bedroom lamp on a night stand
(Figure 3.4). While the person is still asleep, the lamp turns on dimly at about
4:30 a.m. and gradually gets brighter until it reaches full brightness at about
7:00 a.m. However, even at full brightness the lux rating is only 250 lux,
much lower than what we understand is a biologically active intensity.

How does dawn simulation work when the light intensity is so low? In
nature, the day begins not with sudden bright light but with gradual onset
of illumination. We recognize that most people have some awareness of
sunlight in the early morning in the summer, even though the drapes may
be closed and very little light actually reaches the person in bed. Dr George

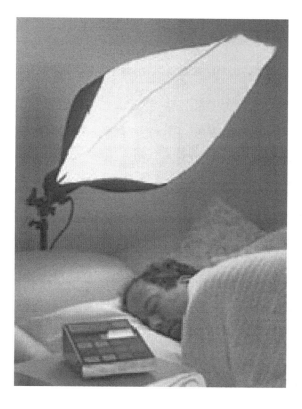

Figure 3.4   A dawn simulator device. Photo courtesy of SphereOne, www.cet.org.

Brainard has shown that low-intensity light (as low as 50 lux) can suppress melatonin secretion under the right conditions, such as when the pupils are dilated with medication. It is possible that the extended darkness during sleep makes the retina more sensitive to light so that even low levels of light can affect circadian rhythms. Once the person wakes and the retina becomes adapted to brighter light, then perhaps a "blast of light" such as that from a bright light box is needed to have the same effects. These are all speculative, however, as we really do not know how dawn simulation works.

Regardless of the explanation, clinical studies have shown an effect of dawn simulation in people with SAD. However, there are very few studies and they have very small sample sizes. In addition, what is not clear is whether this gradual illumination is needed (a "true" dawn simulation) or whether just timing the lights to come on all at once is sufficient. In our clinical experience, patients with SAD only get a mild effect from dawn simulation and do not feel as well as when they are using bright light therapy. However, some patients do find it easier to get up with a dawn simulator and may use it in addition to a light box. Other people simply set their bedroom lights on a timer, as it is much easier to wake up (and stay awake) in a lit room than in a dark one.

Clinical tip

Some people just find it impossible to awake in time to use bright light therapy, or are unable to fit the required 30–60 minutes into their morning routine. For them, dawn simulation offers a good alternative light treatment.

Unproven devices and false claims

There are also many light devices based on unsupported theories. Some of these tout the healing properties of colour therapy, such as specific wavelengths of light or flashing lights without particular consideration for intensity. Presumably, different colours would be prescribed for different symptoms or conditions. While some people may subjectively associate certain colours with a soothing effect, we are not aware of any scientific evidence for coloured or flashing lights having any specific therapeutic effects (except for the circadian effects of blue light; see Chapter 5).

Similarly, there are advertisements for the healing effects of Ott Lights, which emit a much greater amount of ultraviolet wavelengths than other light sources. There is certainly emerging evidence that people do not get enough vitamin D, which is produced by skin exposure to the ultraviolet wavelengths in sunlight and has an important role in calcium absorption and metabolism. This is especially so in the winter when there is little sun exposure. However, our studies and others have shown that the ultraviolet wavelengths are not necessary for the antidepressant effect of light for SAD, and there are also harmful effects of long-term ultraviolet exposure on the eyes, such as cataract formation. Therefore, Ott Lights are not recommended for the treatment of SAD.

Consumers must also be aware that there are many false and misleading claims from some device companies. These usually overstate positive effects and understate potential side effects. For example, we have seen one company market a dim light device with the claim that research had shown this device to be as effective as a bright light box. As evidence, they cited a study in which the dim light and bright light both showed similar results. As discussed in Chapter 5, sometimes studies show negative results – no one study can ever be definitive and it is the totality of evidence that must be evaluated. In this case, the dim light in the study was used as a placebo condition and the researchers concluded that this was a negative study, probably because only a small number of people were studied. The great majority of studies, however, have found dim light to be ineffective, and so this device would not be recommended.

Practical aspects

The cost of a light box or other light device ranges from $100 to $300. Compared to medications, light devices have a higher initial cost. But, since

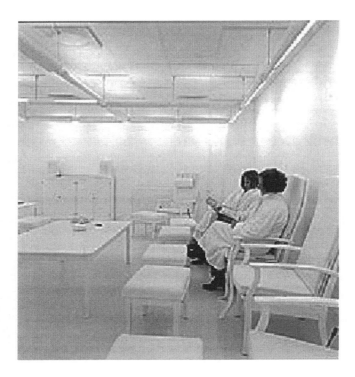

Figure 3.5 Light therapy room in a hospital in Malmo, Sweden. Photo courtesy of Dr. Baba Pendse, Department of Clinical Sciences, Lund University, Sweden.

the cost represents less than 6 months' supply of a newer antidepressant, a light box would be more cost-effective after only one season of use.

Given the cost of a light box, the ideal situation would be to "try before you buy". Some medical supply retailers will rent out light boxes for several weeks so the consumer can determine response, and then apply the cost of rental towards purchase. Some light box companies and retailers offer a money-back guarantee. Some clinics and individual practitioners purchase light boxes to lend out to patients for a brief trial, perhaps for a small handling fee. This system works best if a refundable deposit is taken from the patient, or else the light boxes may not be returned!

People may be able to recover the cost of a light therapy device from their health insurance plan. Although this is often on an individual basis, some insurance companies such as Aetna U.S. Healthcare will reimburse the cost of a light therapy device when medically indicated. Chapter 7 includes a sample letter that we provide to patients with SAD seeking insurance reimbursement.

In Scandinavian countries, some hospitals have "light therapy rooms" where patients receive light therapy in a group format (Figure 3.5). While this appears effective, it does not seem like the most convenient method for a daily treatment. However, in Europe there are also "light cafes" in which people can have a morning cup of coffee and breakfast while receiving their daily dose of light treatment. We think this would be a good idea to import to North America!

Further reading

Desan PH, Weinstein AJ, Michalak EE, Tam EM, Meesters Y, Ruiter MJ, Horn E, Telner J, Iskandar H, Boivin DB, Lam RW. A controlled trial of the Litebook light-emitting diode (LED) light therapy device for treatment of Seasonal Affective Disorder (SAD). *BMC Psychiatry* 2007; **7**:38.

Terman M, Terman JS. Controlled trial of naturalistic dawn simulation and negative air ionization for seasonal affective disorder. *Am J Psychiatry* 2006; **163**:2126–2133.

Rastad C, Ulfberg J, Lindberg P. Light room therapy effective in mild forms of seasonal affective disorder – a randomised controlled study. *J Affect Disord* 2008; **108**:291–296.

Other Treatments, Alone and Combined with Light

There are a number of other treatments for SAD besides light therapy. Some (such as antidepressants) are well-studied while others (such as negative ions) have more limited evidence to support their use. In this chapter, we will briefly review other treatments and describe how they can be used on their own or in combination with light therapy.

Antidepressants

Antidepressants work by modulating neurotransmitters such as serotonin, noradrenaline and/or dopamine. Given that light therapy may also work via effects on these same neurotransmitters, there may be common pathways of action between the two. It is not surprising that antidepressants are also effective in treating SAD.

There are several randomized controlled trials (RCTs) showing the efficacy of selective serotonin reuptake inhibitors (SSRIs) in SAD, including fluoxetine, sertraline and citalopram (Table 4.1; see Pjrek et al., 2005, for a review on this topic). Citalopram has also been used to maintain response after brief (1–2 weeks) treatment with light therapy.

One study deserves particular attention, because it is the largest-ever treatment study of SAD and is the only prevention study using an antidepressant (Modell et al., 2005). Over one thousand patients with seasonal MDD were enrolled in three studies with identical methods. Bupropion-XL 150–300 mg/d was started in the early fall when patients were still well and followed through one winter to determine whether the medication could prevent an episode of winter depression. All three studies showed a significant preventative effect (Figure 4.1). However, it was interesting that there was only a 30% recurrence rate in those patients taking placebo, which suggests that not all people with SAD need prevention treatment.

Open-label studies (i.e., those without placebo control conditions) also suggest that other antidepressants are effective in SAD (Table 4.2). Older medications such as the tricyclic antidepressant desipramine and the monoamine oxidase inhibitor tranylcypromine also show benefit, but these

Table 4.1. Randomized controlled trials of antidepressants in SAD.

Anti-depressant	Author / year[a]	Mode of action	Dose	Comparator	Sample size	Results
Bupropion-XL [Wellbutrin-XL]	Modell et al., 2005	Noradrenaline and dopamine reuptake inhibitor	150–300 mg	Placebo (prevention)	1042	Bupropion > placebo through winter follow-up
Citalopram [Celexa]	Martiny et al., 2004	Selective serotonin reuptake inhibitor	20–40 mg	Placebo (following 1 week of light)	282	Citalopram > placebo through winter follow-up
Fluoxetine [Prozac]	Lam et al., 1995	Selective serotonin reuptake inhibitor	20 mg	Placebo	68	Fluoxetine > placebo (response) after 5 weeks
	Partonen, 1996		20–40 mg	Moclobemide 300–450 mg	32	Fluoxetine = moclobemide after 6 weeks
	Ruhrmann et al., 1998		20 mg	Bright light	40	Fluoxetine = light after 4 weeks
	Lam et al., 2006		20 mg	Bright light	96	Fluoxetine = light after 8 weeks
Moclobemide [Manerix]	Lingjaerde et al., 1993	Reversible inhibitor of monoamine oxidase-A	400 mg	Placebo	34	Moclobemide = placebo after 3 weeks
Sertraline [Zoloft]	Moscovitch et al., 2004	Selective serotonin reuptake inhibitor	50–200 mg	Placebo	187	Sertraline > placebo after 8 weeks

[a] For full references, see Pjrek et al., 2005.

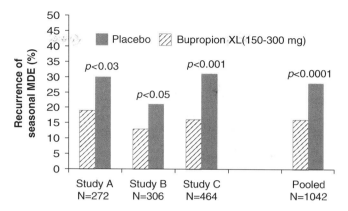

Figure 4.1 Bupropion-XL for prevention of seasonal major depressive episodes (MDEs), Modell et al., 2005. Figure adapted from Westrin Å, Lam RW. Seasonal affective disorder: A clinical update. *Ann Clin Psychiatry* 2007; 19:239–246.

medications are associated with more side effects and some require dietary and drug restrictions. A particularly interesting new antidepressant is agomelatine, which acts as an agonist of melatonin-1 (MT_1) and melatonin-2 (MT_2) receptors and an antagonist of the serotonin 2C ($5\text{-}HT_{2C}$) receptor. Agomelatine is effective in nonseasonal depression, but also appears effective in SAD.

Clinical example

> Ted had a good response to light therapy initially, but found in subsequent years that it had less effect. After trials of different antidepressants, he found that he tolerated bupropion the best. He now starts using light therapy each autumn, and adds bupropion if he notices breakthrough symptoms.

There has also been some interest in medications that are not specifically antidepressants. Modafanil is a "wake-promoting" medication used for the treatment of narcolepsy (Table 4.2). It is not a stimulant drug, but it has been shown in one open study to reduce fatigue in those suffering from SAD,

| Table 4.2. | Uncontrolled, open-label studies of medications in SAD. |

Medication	Author / year	Mode of action	Dose	Sample size	Results
Agomelatine [Valdoxan]	Pjrek et al., 2007a	MT_1 and MT_2 agonist; $5-HT_{2C}$ antagonist	25–50 mg	37	70% remission after 14 weeks
Duloxetine [Cymbalta]	Pjrek et al., 2008	Serotonin and noradrenaline reuptake inhibitor		26	77% remission after 8 weeks
Escitalopram [Cipralex, Lexapro]	Pjrek et al., 2007b	Allosteric serotonin reuptake inhibitor	10–20 mg	20	85% remission after 8 weeks
Mirtazapine [Remeron]	Hesselmann et al., 1999	α_2-Adrenergic agonist; $5-HT_{2C}$ antagonist	30–45 mg	8	75% response after 6 weeks
Modafinil [Provigil]	Lundt, 2004	Wake-promoting		12	67% response after 8 weeks
Reboxetine [Edronax]	Hilger et al., 2001	Noradrenaline reuptake inhibitor		16	69% remission after 6 weeks

and may be helpful in treating residual symptoms. Hypnotic medications (benzodiazepine and non-benzodiazepine drugs) can be used to provide short-term relief from depression-induced insomnia. Usually they can be discontinued when the depression responds to treatment.

Many patients whose winter depression responds to antidepressants can stop the medication in the spring/summer when they are in natural remission. They then restart taking the antidepressant in the early fall before onset of symptoms. Other patients find it easier to stay on the medication year-round, particularly if they have few side effects.

How to choose between antidepressants and light therapy

How does light therapy compare to antidepressants? We conducted the first large-sample RCT to answer this question. The CAN-SAD study involved 96 patients with SAD in five centres across Canada (Lam et al., 2006). To balance expectations of treatment, patients all took a pill and used a fluorescent light box for 30 minutes each morning for 8 weeks. Half the sample was randomized to placebo pill and active bright white

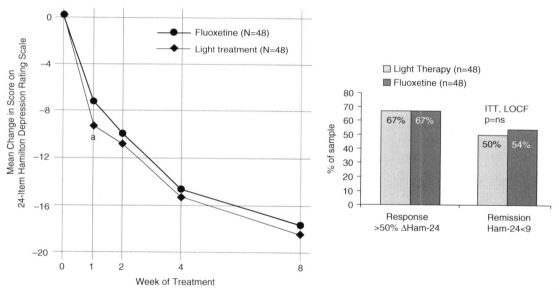

aSignificantly greater improvement in the first week of treatment for those receiving light therapy relative to those receiving fluoxetine (t=2.1, df=94, p<0.05).

Figure 4.2   Summary results from the CAN-SAD RCT of light therapy versus fluoxetine in SAD. ITT=Intent to Treat, LOCF=Last Observation Carried Forward, ns=not significant. Figure adapted from: Lam RW, Levitt AJ, Levitan RD, Enns MW, Morehouse R, Michalak EE, Tam EM. The Can-SAD study: a randomized controlled trial of the effectiveness of light therapy and fluoxetine in patients with winter seasonal affective disorder. *Am J Psychiatry* 2006; 163:805–812.

light (10,000 lux) and the other half to fluoxetine (Prozac) 20 mg and placebo dim light (300 lux). The results showed that both treatments worked equally well, although the patients using bright light had a faster response (at 1 week) than those taking fluoxetine (Figure 4.2). At 8 weeks, the clinical response rate was 67% for both conditions, while the remission rate was 50% for bright light and 54% for fluoxetine. Both treatments were also well tolerated, although more of the fluoxetine-treated group experienced side effects of agitation, sleep disturbance, and palpitations.

Given that both treatments are similarly effective, the choice of treatment depends on other factors, including patient preference (Table 4.3). While light therapy can be very effective and well tolerated, it can be too time-consuming and inconvenient for some patients. The cost of a light box is about the same as a season's worth of the newer antidepressants, but it becomes cost-effective when used season after season. However, many insurance plans will cover medications but may not cover a light box. Still others may have relative contraindications for one or the other treatment.

Table 4.3. **Factors to consider when deciding between light therapy and antidepressants for SAD. Note that none of these factors is an absolute indication.**

Light therapy favoured if:	Medications favoured if:
• Personal preference is for light therapy	• Personal preference is for medication
• Motivated and able to follow light therapy protocol	• Not motivated or unable to follow light therapy protocol
• Medications are relatively contraindicated (e.g., illness, pregnancy, breast-feeding)	• Light therapy is relatively contraindicated (e.g., retinal disease)
• Atypical symptoms are prominent	• Melancholic symptoms are prominent
• Medications give intolerable side effects	• Light therapy gives intolerable side effects
• Able to afford light device	• Unable to afford light device, but medications are covered

Combining antidepressants and light therapy

Sometimes, light therapy provides a good partial response but falls short of achieving full remission. At other times, the effect of light therapy seems to subside over the years. In these cases, combining light with medications may be indicated. Indeed, naturalistic follow-up studies show that many patients use both light and antidepressants, which is why it is surprising that there are no studies (yet) of combination treatment in SAD (although there are studies of combination treatment in nonseasonal MDD).

In general, people who are interested in light therapy tend to prefer "natural" approaches and are wary of medications. Thus, they may need a lot of education and discussion before starting an antidepressant. One situation that may warrant combining both treatments from the beginning would be a patient suffering from severe depression. Light therapy may produce a more rapid response, in some people, but starting an antidepressant at the same time will not delay medication response if light therapy is not effective. It is also possible that the combined treatment may have synergistic effects.

There are no absolute contraindications to using antidepressants with light therapy. In our experience, we have found that patients can often manage on lower doses of antidepressants when combined with light, compared to taking the medication alone.

Cognitive behavioural therapy

Because SAD seems related to the environmental stress of winter and since most of the initial theories involved biological processes, the psychological aspects of SAD have only recently attracted scientific attention. Several studies have shown that SAD, like other types of depression, is associated with automatic negative thoughts and maladaptive attitudes and assumptions. Dr Michael Young first proposed the dual vulnerability hypothesis for SAD. This theory states that the seasonal changes in physiological symptoms trigger negative cognitions that lead to rumination and depressive symptoms and behaviours. If true, it seems reasonable to address these negative cognitions to treat SAD.

Cognitive behavioural therapy (CBT) is an evidence-based psychotherapy for depression that seeks to help people identify the negative thinking patterns and dysfunctional behaviours associated with depression, and learn practical techniques to deal with them. Dr Kelly Rohan and colleagues have taken this CBT approach and tailored it specifically to SAD. In addition, they believe that people can apply these techniques to anticipate winter changes in mood and physical symptoms, and thereby prevent problems in subsequent winters. Initial studies using this CBT approach were encouraging and further larger studies are in progress. One study showed that combining CBT with light therapy did not show better results than either treatment alone in the short term; however, on naturalistic follow-up, the people treated with the combination had better outcomes in the subsequent winter.

> ### Clinical tip
>
> Dr Kelly Rohan has recently published a treatment manual for clinicians who want to use tailored CBT for SAD (see "Further reading"). A client workbook is also available.

Herbal and nutriceutical treatments

Melatonin is a neurohormone that is integral to the sleep–wake cycle and possibly involved in the circadian rhythm etiology of SAD (see Chapter 5). Initial studies using pharmacological doses of melatonin had no effect in SAD. However, Dr Alfred Lewy has been studying lower, more physiological doses of melatonin that can induce circadian phase shifts similar to bright light. Using this phase-shifting approach, his group found that appropriately timed (in the late afternoon) doses of melatonin had an antidepressant effect in some patients with SAD.

Tryptophan is a naturally occurring amino acid that is a precursor for serotonin, which is a key neurotransmitter in SAD. Tryptophan was found to be useful in an open-label study to boost a partial response to light therapy, and in a controlled trial as a stand-alone treatment with a response similar to evening light therapy. Tryptophan can be a useful second-step in treatment after light therapy, especially in cases where the patient is reluctant to use "non-natural" products. We suggest using 1 gram three times a day. Side effects can include stomach upset, especially when taken on an empty stomach, so we recommend taking it with meals.

Clinical example

Clara did not want to use anything unnatural in her treatment regimen, and so refused any suggestion of antidepressants. However, she was agreeable to trying tryptophan with her light therapy. She found the combination improved her symptoms.

Another treatment often preferred for its natural properties is St John's wort, also known as hypericum after its active ingredient. It is a plant extract that has been shown in many studies to be effective for mild to moderate nonseasonal depression. It may be helpful in SAD, but it also has photosensitizing effects and so should be used cautiously if combined with bright light.

There is no good evidence that vitamins are beneficial for SAD. Cyanocobalamin (vitamin B12) can affect circadian rhythms, but it was not effective in SAD. There has been general interest in vitamin D because its production requires sun exposure (specifically the ultraviolet wavelengths of sunlight) and many people do not produce enough in the winter. Vitamin D supplementation (at least 1000 International Units per day) is recommended for general bone health, but supplementation does not appear to improve mood in the winter.

Other treatments (negative ions, exercise)

Negative ions have long been touted as improving mood and well-being, but some recent studies have shown that they may also be effective in treating SAD and other types of depression. These preliminary results need to be confirmed in larger studies before negative ion treatment can be recommended for general clinical use. However, the use of negative ions is attractive because it has few side effects and is very convenient because it does not require any special activity. Like dawn simulation, negative ions can even be used during sleep! The scientific studies used special ion generators that produce high-density negative ions – not the usual low-density negative ion generators that you can buy for home use. The Center for Environmental Therapeutics (www.cet.org) has more information on how to obtain high-density negative ion generators.

Exercise has also been shown to have mild antidepressant effects. It has the advantage of being a "natural" treatment often sought by people with SAD and can complement light therapy. Exercise by itself is usually not potent enough to be a sole treatment for SAD, although one study reported that 60 minutes of aerobic exercise a day was as effective as light therapy. It also requires motivation and discipline to integrate exercise into a depressed patient's schedule. The best results are usually obtained when an exercise program is started in the fall to help prevent a winter episode, since it is very hard to start exercising when in the midst of a depression.

Clinical example

Susan had a partial response to light therapy, and wanted to use exercise as adjunctive treatment. However, she was a student and, between her course work and her depression-induced low energy and motivation, she was unable to keep up a regular exercise program. Her breakthrough came during the Christmas holidays, when she could devote time and energy to make exercise a part of her weekly routine. She was then able to continue her exercise routine even after school restarted, and she achieved full remission with this combination.

Clinical example

Roger has been managing well each winter using a combination of light therapy and jogging. However, this year he sustained an ankle injury and was unable to continue his usual jogging. To his chagrin, the light therapy alone was not enough to keep his winter depression at bay, and he began to experience a return of depressive symptoms.

Further reading

Lam RW, Levitt AJ, Levitan RD, Enns MW, Morehouse R, Michalak EE, Tam EM. The Can-SAD study: a randomized controlled trial of the effectiveness of light therapy and fluoxetine in patients with winter seasonal affective disorder. *Am J Psychiatry* 2006; **163**:805–812.

Lewy AJ, Emens J, Jackman A, Yuhas K. Circadian uses of melatonin in humans. *Chronobiol Int* 2006; **23**:403–412.

Modell JG, Rosenthal NE, Harriett AE, Krishen A, Asgharian A, Foster VJ, Metz A, Rockett CB, Wightman DS. Seasonal affective disorder and its prevention by anticipatory treatment with bupropion XL. *Biol Psychiatry* 2005; **58**:658–667.

Pjrek E, Winkler D, Kasper S. Pharmacotherapy of seasonal affective disorder. *CNS Spectr* 2005 Aug;**10**(8):664–669.

Rohan KJ. *Coping with the Seasons. A Cognitive Behavioral Approach for Seasonal Affective Disorder.* Therapist and Client Workbook Guides. London: Oxford University Press, 2008.

Rohan KJ, Roecklein KA, Tierney Lindsey K, Johnson LG, Lippy RD, Lacy TJ, Barton FB. A randomized controlled trial of cognitive-behavioral therapy, light therapy, and their combination for seasonal affective disorder. *J Consult Clin Psychol* 2007; **75**:489–500.

Teicher MH, Glod CA, Oren DA, Schwartz PJ, Luetke C, Brown C, Rosenthal NE. The phototherapy light visor: more to it than meets the eye. *Am J Psychiatry* 1995; **152**:1197–202.

Terman M, Terman JS. Controlled trial of naturalistic dawn simulation and negative air ionization for seasonal affective disorder. *Am J Psychiatry* 2006; **163**:2126–2133.

Young MA, Watel LG, Lahmeyer HW, Eastman CI. The temporal onset of individual symptoms in winter depression: differentiating underlying mechanisms. *J Affect Disord* 1991; **22**:191–197.

Effectiveness and Mechanism of Action

There have been over 100 studies of light therapy for SAD and other conditions, but some studies are of higher quality than others. In today's evidence-based medical environment, and especially when third-party payers are demanding evidence to support funding for treatments, it is important to assess the effectiveness of light therapy in a rigorous way. In this chapter, we identify some of the issues with evaluating effectiveness, especially for non-pharmacological treatments, review the specific evidence for effectiveness of light therapy, and summarize the major theories for its mechanism of action.

How to measure effectiveness of treatments

Why can't you evaluate effectiveness by simply using a treatment and measuring improvement? The answer is because people may feel better for many reasons that have nothing to do with the treatment. For example, symptoms may fluctuate in severity or spontaneously improve, patients may be relieved at being treated or respond to the investigator's enthusiasm, there may be changes in their environment (e.g., a change from cloudy to sunny weather, spending more time outdoors), the investigator may be biased to over-rate improvement, and so forth. To properly evaluate a treatment requires attention to controlling for these many sources of bias.

The highest-quality treatment study in medicine is a randomized controlled trial (RCT) with a double-blind placebo control condition. Randomization is essential to minimize bias because it balances out any identified or unknown factors that may affect outcome. For example, it is possible that women are more likely to sit in front of a light box than men. Randomization ensures that an equal number of men and women are balanced between those on placebo and those in the active treatment so that there is no bias in rating outcome. A placebo condition is important because it negates any bias due to non-specific factors (such as sitting quietly for 30 minutes) that can affect outcome. Double-blind refers to the situation where neither the patient nor the doctor (or person rating their symptoms) knows whether the patient is taking the active treatment or the placebo. This is important because differential expectations may influence outcomes, e.g., if the doctor knows the patient is taking a placebo, he or she may be less enthusiastic and treat the patient differently.

Sample size is also an important consideration. Larger sample sizes provide more statistical confidence about the results, particularly when the results are negative. The results from small studies are more likely to be influenced by random and non-random biases, and so require confirmation by replication. Multi-centre studies are usually preferred over single-centre because the results are more generalizable to other samples and settings.

However, some RCTs may have positive results while others have negative ones. How do we evaluate the results of many studies with conflicting results? One method is having an expert review the results to give an expert opinion. However, an expert can also be biased and it is often not clear how individual studies are weighted in the expert opinion. Consequently, there has been a shift to replace the subjective expert opinion with meta-analysis, a statistical technique used to combine results from many studies to arrive at one overall conclusion. Meta-analysis addresses issues such as bias and sample size to provide a quantitative assessment of treatment effectiveness. A well-conducted meta-analysis is now regarded as one of the highest-quality types of evidence to evaluate the efficacy of treatments.

Another point to remember is that results can be statistically significant and yet may not be clinically relevant. For example, a study may show that a 1-point average difference in depression scores is statistically significant, but most clinicians would not consider that difference to be clinically important. Good-quality studies should include clinical measures of response in addition to outcomes on rating scales.

The placebo effect: myths and realities

The placebo effect is arguably the most important issue for treatment studies of "subjective" conditions such as depression. Many people mistakenly believe the placebo effect to be "all in your head". In reality, it describes all the non-specific elements in a study that contribute to improvement, in contrast to any specific effect of a treatment. For example, in clinical trials, patients attend regularly scheduled clinic visits, learn about their illness, monitor their symptoms, and interact socially with the research team. Many of these non-specific elements are included in "behavioural activation", which itself is an effective treatment for depression. Patients also often experience renewed hope and enthusiasm about a new treatment. Therefore, it is not surprising that people who are depressed feel better during a clinical trial, even if they are taking a placebo.

It is easy to incorporate a double-blind placebo condition when studying a new drug because a placebo pill can be used which is identical in appearance and taste but contains no active drug. It is much more difficult to design a double-blind placebo for a non-medication treatment such as light therapy. A good placebo condition must control for all the potential non-specific effects of light therapy such as getting up at the same time each morning, sitting quietly for a period, using a "high-tech" device, and so on. However, light cannot be disguised so other creative solutions must be found. Many studies used so-called dim light of 300–500 lux as a control condition for active bright light. The advantage of dim light as a placebo is that an identical light apparatus can be used. The disadvantage is that you can never be sure that the dim light "dose" is not therapeutically active in some patients. In addition, patients may be aware that their light is dim and so may not be truly "blind" to treatment assignment.

Another creative placebo condition used in studies is a negative ion generator. The advantage of this non-light placebo is that it can be used in exactly the same way as light, but there is no worry about a low-dose light effect. Negative ions are a plausible treatment for SAD because there is public perception that negative ions have beneficial health effects. In several studies, the placebo negative ion generator had a power light and produced a nice humming sound but, unknown to the patient, was deactivated so that no negative ions were generated! Other studies used a generator that produced low-density negative ions, which are not known to have any therapeutic effects, as the placebo condition.

| Table 5.1. | Meta-analyses examining effectiveness of light therapy. |

Author	Inclusion criteria	No. of included studies	Main findings
Terman et al., 1989	Open trials and RCTs	29 studies	• Bright light showed higher remission rates than dim light. • Early morning exposure had higher remission rates than evening and midday.
Lee and Chan, 1999	Open trials and RCTs	39 studies	• Bright light was superior to dim light.
Thompson, 2001	RCTs	14 studies	• Bright light was superior to control conditions. • Morning exposure was superior to other times of the day.
Golden et al., 2005	RCTs	8 studies (light treatment) 4 studies (dawn stimulation)	• Bright light and dawn simulation were both superior to control conditions. • Morning exposure was superior to other times of the day.

The evidence for light therapy in SAD

An early meta-analysis conducted by Drs Michael and Jiuan Terman summarized the first 5 years of light therapy studies (Table 5.1). This pooled analysis found that bright light was effective and that morning light exposure was superior to other times of the day. However, the included studies were criticized for their small samples, short treatment durations, and lack of adequate placebo controls and blinding. Many of these first studies were designed to examine biological aspects of SAD or mechanisms of action of light therapy, and not primarily to evaluate therapeutic effects.

Several larger, better-quality RCTs were conducted in the early to mid-1990s, and three were published in 1998 in the same issue of Archives of General Psychiatry, the top-ranked psychiatric journal. Dr Terman and colleagues studied a 10,000 lux light box given for 30 minutes in the morning or the evening for 2–4 weeks, versus a negative ion generator. In one condition, the negative ion generator produced low-density negative ions (the placebo) while in another, high-density negative ions were produced. They found that the bright light was superior to the low-density negative ion placebo, and that morning light was superior to evening light. In addition, the high-density negative ion condition was also superior to placebo, and not different from the bright light.

Dr Charmane Eastman and colleagues examined 5,000 lux given for one hour, either in the morning or the evening for 5 weeks, versus a negative ion generator that, unknown to the patient, was inactivated so no negative

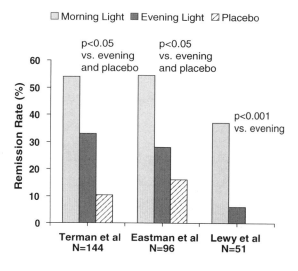

Figure 5.1 Summary results from three high-quality RCTs of light therapy for SAD.

ions were produced. They also found that, on measures of clinical response, bright light was more effective than the placebo condition. Again, morning light exposure was superior to evening on several of the outcome measures.

In the third study, Dr Alfred Lewy and colleagues examined 5,000 lux for 45 minutes of morning versus evening exposure for 4 weeks. A placebo condition was not used. However, the morning light was significantly superior to evening light, suggesting that not all the benefits could be explained by placebo (since one would not expect differential placebo response rates based on different timing, unless the patients expected one to work better than the other).

In summary, these three studies had larger sample sizes and higher-quality clinical trial methods including closer attention to placebo and non-specific effects of light treatment. The results were consistent: bright light was superior to plausible placebo conditions and morning exposure was superior to evening. The bright morning light treatment produced remission rates of about 55%. Together these studies offer strong support for the efficacy of light therapy.

Since these studies were published, some negative studies have also been reported. For example, a study conducted in Scotland examined people who were identified in a community survey as having SAD and randomized them to bright or dim light conditions (Wileman et al., 2001). They found no differences in response in any of the outcome measures. However, this is the only study to use a community survey to recruit patients, rather than using patients seeking help. It is possible that these patients were different (e.g., less severe, less motivated for treatment) from patients in other light therapy studies. In addition, patients were allowed to use the light as long as they wanted, and at whatever time of day they wanted. Therefore, many people may not have been using an effective light treatment method.

Several recent meta-analyses of light therapy have also been conducted (Table 5.1). These various meta-analyses have used different criteria for selecting studies, which is why the included studies range from 8 to

39 studies. One study used the rigorous methodology of the Cochrane Collaboration, an international scientific society dedicated to evidence-based medicine and meta-analyses (Thompson, 2001). This meta-analysis of 14 RCTs found that bright light was more efficacious than control conditions. Another meta-analysis, commissioned by the American Psychiatric Association, used even stricter inclusion criteria so that only eight RCTs were included (Golden et al., 2005). It also concluded that bright light demonstrated significant effects compared with placebo conditions. Both meta-analyses also found that morning light exposure was superior to other times.

In summary, numerous RCTs and other treatment studies have shown that bright light therapy is effective in SAD. These findings are confirmed by meta-analyses. The studies also consistently find that morning exposure is better than other times of the day. We can conclude from this body of research that morning light therapy is a well-validated, evidence-based treatment for SAD. In fact, light therapy is recognized as a first-line treatment for SAD in clinical practice guidelines for depression produced by several international professional and scientific societies.

How does light therapy work?

The mechanism of action by which light exerts its antidepressant effects has been intimately tied to the study of the causes of SAD. We know that light is the strongest synchronizer of the circadian system and that exposure to bright light has predictable effects on human circadian rhythms. What we do not know, however, is whether the circadian effects of light explain the antidepressant effects in SAD and other conditions. Several recent reviews have detailed the studies examining the pathophysiology of SAD and the mechanism of action of light therapy (see "Further reading"). We will briefly review the effects of light on the human circadian system and the main theories about how light therapy works.

Circadian rhythms: a primer

Circadian means "daily", so circadian rhythms refer to the daily cycles of activity, hormones and behaviours. Most circadian rhythms are controlled by a biological clock located in the suprachiasmatic nucleus (SCN) of the hypothalamus. Light entering the eye acts as a zeitgeber (synchronizer) of the SCN pacemaker. There is a direct neural pathway, the retinohypothalamic

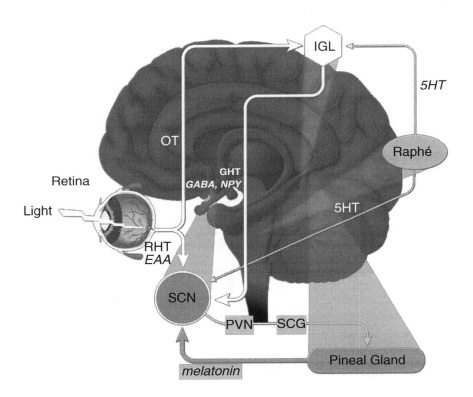

Figure 5.2   The human circadian system. Figure taken from Wirz-Justice A. Biological rhythms in mood disorders. In: Bloom FE, Kupfer DJ (eds). *Psychopharmacology: the Fourth Generation of Progress*. New York: Raven Press, 1995, pp. 999–1017. Abbreviations: RHT = retinohypothalamic tract; SCN = suprachiasmatic nucleus; PVN = paraventricular nucleus; SCG = superior cervical ganglion; OT = optic tract; IGL = intergeniculate leaflet; 5HT = 5-hydroxytryptamine (serotonin); GABA = gamma aminobutyric acid; NPY = neuropeptide Y.

tract, leading from the retina to the SCN. From there, a more complicated pathway leads from the SCN to the pineal gland to control melatonin secretion (Figure 5.2).

There are several important features that describe circadian rhythms: period, amplitude, and phase (Figure 5.3). Phase is usually indicated by the time of a particular point in the cycle, e.g., the peak of cortisol secretion or the core body temperature minimum.

- Period – the time interval between two cycles.
- Amplitude – the difference between the peak and midpoint or trough of a cycle.
- Phase – the relationship of the cycle to external time (or to another type of rhythm).
- Phase shift – a change in the relationship of the cycle to external time (or to another type of rhythm).

Measuring circadian rhythms is not easy because sampling must be done over a 24-hour period, sometimes for many days or weeks. This is often technically difficult because multiple blood samples or temperature readings are required. There are also many factors that affect endogenous circadian rhythms, such as ambient light exposure, activity, digestion, etc. Some of the best indicators of circadian rhythms include core body temperature,

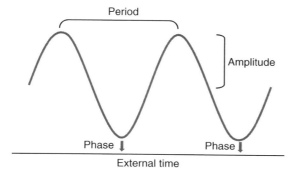

Figure 5.3 Graphical representation of circadian rhythm measures.

melatonin onset, and polysomnography (sleep EEG). The dim light melatonin onset (DLMO) describes the time that melatonin begins to be secreted at night when it is sampled under dim light conditions. The DLMO is a particularly important circadian measure because it is not affected by many environmental factors and can be more easily obtained than others. The circadian phase of an individual can be determined by sampling plasma melatonin every half hour during the evening. Newer techniques can measure the melatonin concentration in saliva, which is much more convenient than taking blood samples.

Melatonin secretion is also suppressed by light. In animals, even relatively dim room light (<300 lux) can suppress melatonin secretion and phase-shift circadian rhythms (see next section). Interestingly, human melatonin secretion was not suppressed by room light and human circadian rhythms could not be shifted in the same way as animal, leading some early investigators to suggest that humans had evolved past the point of dependence on the light–dark cycle.

Obviously we are much closer to our animal relatives than thought, because in 1980 it was shown that human melatonin could be suppressed by light after all, but much brighter light was required. Dr Alfred Lewy and his colleagues at the U.S. National Institute of Mental Health found that bright light of at least 1,500 lux was required to suppress human melatonin under natural conditions. Circadian studies were re-done using this much brighter light intensity and confirmed that human circadian rhythms could predictably be phase-shifted, similarly to how a much dimmer light shifted rhythms in animals. It was this observation that contributed to the theory that SAD could be treated using bright light.

Phase-shifting effects of light

The effect of bright light on the circadian system depends on when the light is given in the cycle. This can be illustrated by the phase-response curve, in which bright light is presented at different points in the circadian cycle and the resultant change in phase is plotted. In the middle of the circadian cycle

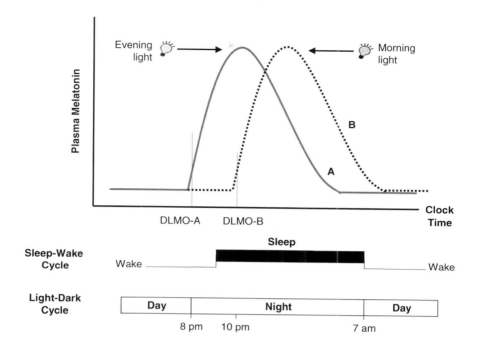

Figure 5.4 Phase shifts with morning and evening light exposure, as measured by dim light melatonin onset (DLMO). Figure adapted from Sohn CH, Lam RW. Update on the biology of seasonal affective disorder. *CNS Spectr* 2005; 10:635–646.

(midday/afternoon in humans), there is a circadian "dead zone" in which bright light does not shift the rhythm. Light given in the early part of the cycle (early morning in humans) results in a phase-advance of the rhythm (i.e., the circadian rhythm moves earlier in external clock time), while light given in the later part of the cycle (evening in humans) results in a phase delay (i.e., the circadian rhythm moves later in external clock time) (Figure 5.4).

This figure illustrates phase-shifting using the melatonin secretion curve as an example of a circadian rhythm and the DLMO as a measure of circadian phase. Subject "A" (solid line) is a "normal" person whose circadian phase is indicated by the clock time represented as DLMO-A. Subject "B" (dotted line) represents a person with SAD. B is phase-delayed relative to A because DLMO-B occurs at a later clock time than DLMO-A. If B is exposed to morning bright light, B's melatonin rhythm shifts so that DLMO-B moves earlier in time towards the "normal" DLMO-A. This represents a corrective phase advance of circadian rhythms.

Conversely, if A is exposed to bright light in the late evening, the melatonin rhythm shifts in the opposite direction (from the solid-line curve towards the dotted-line curve) and on subsequent nights A's DLMO shifts to the later time indicated by DLMO-B. This illustrates a phase delay of circadian rhythms.

Interestingly, the magnitude of the phase shift increases as the bright light stimulus is timed closer to the lowest point of the core body temperature rhythm, which for "normal" people occurs about 4 a.m. That is, bright light at 3:30 a.m. produces a larger phase delay than light given at 3:00 a.m., which produces a larger delay than light given at 2:30 a.m. Conversely, bright light at 4:30 a.m. results in a larger phase advance than a light stimulus at 5:00 a.m., which produces a larger advance than light given at 5:30 a.m. Therefore, the phase-shifting effect of bright light rapidly changes from a maximal phase delay to a maximal phase advance at an inflection point around 4:00 a.m.

This peculiar property of the phase-response curve is essential to understanding the use of bright light to treat circadian sleep–wake disorders. The important point is that to correct phase abnormalities, bright light must be appropriately timed relative to an individual's inflection point, which depends on their circadian phase. For example, if someone has phase-delayed sleep disorder, the treatment is a corrective phase advance by morning light exposure (Figure 5.4). We can say that, for most people, light in the early morning around 6:00 a.m. will predictably phase-advance, while light in the late evening (after 11pm) will result in phase delays. However, this can vary by as much as 4 hours from person to person. Without knowing their inflection point, it is possible to mis-time the light exposure and shift the rhythm in the opposite direction!

Given this inter-individual variability, it is very challenging to properly time light exposure without a measurement of circadian phase. Unfortunately, it is still very difficult to measure circadian phase in patients in clinical settings. In future, salivary sampling of melatonin may become more widely available so it will be more feasible to measure the DLMO and properly time light exposure in people with circadian rhythm disorders.

Photoperiod theory

The rationale for this theory is that seasonal changes in animal behaviour reflect the photoperiod – the length of the day – which is longer in summer and shorter in winter. Many animals "sense" the photoperiod via the duration of melatonin secretion, since melatonin is only secreted in the night. Extending the photoperiod by exposing the animal to artificial light at dawn and dusk changes winter behaviours to summer ones.

The photoperiod theory of SAD is supported by studies showing that the prevalence of SAD increases with higher latitude (with corresponding shorter photoperiods in winter), but is not correlated to weather variables such as temperature, barometric pressure, rainfall, snowfall, etc. The first study of light therapy tested this theory by exposing patients with SAD to bright light (2,500 lux) for 2 hours in the early morning (before a winter dawn) and 2 hours in the late evening (after winter dusk). This photoperiod extension resulted in improvement in symptoms of SAD.

However, subsequent studies have shown that photoperiod extension is not necessary for the therapeutic effect of light in SAD. For example, light at other times of the day appeared to have some antidepressant effects, and even a short duration of light exposure in the morning was effective. Therefore, the photoperiod hypothesis was felt to be disproved. However, more recent studies have resurrected the photoperiod extension hypothesis, as it may relate to melatonin secretion.

Phase-shift theory

The phase-shift hypothesis has been extensively studied and reflects the known effects of light on circadian rhythms. In this hypothesis, SAD is regarded as a problem with delayed circadian phase, similar to travelling east across many time zones. The internal clock of patients with SAD is "out of synch" and delayed relative to external clock time (or to other internal rhythms such as sleep–wake), resulting in symptoms similar to jet lag (sleep–wake problems, fatigue, poor concentration, depressed mood). To correct this phase delay, bright light must be appropriately timed and given in the early morning.

In support of this theory, many studies have shown that morning light is superior to light at other times of the day. In addition, some evidence suggests that the improvement in depression scores is correlated with the magnitude of circadian phase shift with light. Other studies show that shifting circadian phase using non-light methods, such as with melatonin, is also effective in treating SAD.

However, there are also many studies that do not support the phase-delay hypothesis. Studies using the most rigorous measurements of circadian rhythms have not consistently shown phase-delayed rhythms in patients with SAD. In addition, several treatment studies did not find any correlation between phase shift and clinical improvement.

In summary, there are many attractive features of the phase-shift hypothesis, and it is clear that morning light shifts circadian rhythms, but it is still not clear whether this is related to the therapeutic effects of light. It is possible that this theory explains the mode of action for at least a subset of patients, which is why we have recommended optimizing the timing of light therapy based on the phase-shift hypothesis in patients who are not showing response to the simplified light protocol (see Chapter 2).

Neurotransmitter theory

Given the inconsistent evidence for circadian mechanisms of light therapy, what other theories can explain the therapeutic effects of light? There is a great deal of evidence implicating neurotransmitters such as serotonin, dopamine, and noradrenaline in the pathophysiology of MDD and to the mechanism of action of all antidepressant drugs, so it is not surprising that this theory has also been studied in SAD. Of interest is that serotonin is the only neurotransmitter that shows a distinctive seasonal pattern in metabolism, even in healthy people. For example, 5-HIAA, a metabolite of serotonin, is lowest in the cerebrospinal fluid in winter/spring, and a measure of serotonin turnover is also lowest during that time of year. A number of studies have shown evidence for serotonin dysregulation in patients with SAD, with "normalization" following light therapy.

However, while these studies are interesting, they only show correlations and cannot address causation. One never knows whether biological changes that occur following treatment are directly caused by that treatment or whether they simply result from improved mood. Several studies have used an interesting technique called monoamine depletion as a more direct test of whether neurotransmitters are involved in the mechanism of action of light therapy.

One such technique induces rapid depletion of tryptophan, the amino acid precursor of serotonin. By ingesting large amounts of other amino acids, blood levels of tryptophan can be temporarily reduced to 20% of normal levels within 5 hours. In animal studies and human imaging studies, this degree of tryptophan depletion leads to corresponding reductions in serotonin in the brain. If we believe that SAD is associated with reduced levels of serotonin and that light therapy acts by increasing these levels, then we would expect that reducing serotonin by tryptophan depletion would reverse the effect of light therapy. In several studies this was found to be the case.

Similar studies have been done using catecholamine depletion with alpha-methyl-para-tyrosine, which depletes both noradrenaline and dopamine. The catecholamine depletion also reversed the antidepressant effects of light therapy, and made SAD patients more depressed in the summer time. These studies give good evidence that the therapeutic effects of light therapy are related to neurotransmitters.

The importance of these studies is that they provide a rationale for the use of light therapy in other conditions where modifying neurotransmitter levels may be helpful, and also for the use of light as adjunctive to other treatments that affect neurotransmitters (e.g., in combination with antidepressant medications).

The dual vulnerability hypothesis

There are still many inconsistent or discrepant results in the biological and psychological study of SAD and the mechanism of action of light therapy. This suggests that there is much more heterogeneity than was originally expected when SAD and light treatment were first described. The dual vulnerability hypothesis was first proposed by Dr Michael Young to explain the dimensional nature of seasonality and its relationship to SAD. The hypothesis states that SAD results from two processes: a physiological process that produces the characteristic seasonal vegetative symptoms, and a depressive cognitive process that leads to an MDE and the diagnosis of SAD. We have modified and extended this hypothesis to suggest that people have differential loadings on a seasonal factor (such as circadian phase delay) and a depressive factor (such as negative cognitions, or serotonergic dysfunction) that may explain the different presentations and variants of SAD and seasonality. Presumably, light may also have differential effects (both mechanistically and therapeutically) on these two factors, which could explain the variable response to light and its usefulness in both circadian and non-circadian conditions.

Further reading

Effectiveness

American Psychiatric Association. Practice Guideline for the Treatment of Patients with Major Depressive Disorder (Revision, April, 2000). *Am J Psychiatry* 2000; **157**(4) (Supplement): 31. www.psych.org

Bauer M, Whybrow PC, Angst J, Versiani M, Moller H-J. World Federation of Societies of Biological Psychiatry (WFSBP) guidelines for biological treatment of unipolar depressive disorders, Part 1: Acute and continuation treatment of major depressive disorder. *World J Biol Psychiatry* 2002; **3**:5–43.

Eastman CI, Young MA, Fogg LF, Liu L, Meaden PM. Bright light treatment of winter depression: a placebo-controlled trial. *Arch Gen Psychiatry* 1998; **55**:883–889.

Golden RN, Gaynes BN, Ekstrom RD, Hamer RM, Jacobsen FM, Suppes T, Wisner KL, Nemeroff CB. The efficacy of light therapy in the treatment of mood disorders: a review and meta-analysis of the evidence. *Am J Psychiatry* 2005; **162**:656–662.

Kennedy SH, Lam RW, Cohen NL, Ravindran AV. Clinical guidelines for the treatment of depressive disorders. IV. Pharmacotherapy and other biological treatments. *Can J Psychiatry* 2001; **46**(Supplement 1):38S–58S. www.cpa-apc.org

Lam RW, Levitt AJ (eds). *Canadian Consensus Guidelines for the Treatment of Seasonal Affective Disorder*. Vancouver, BC; Clinical & Academic Publishing, 1999. Available at www.UBCsad.ca

Lee TM, Chan CC. Dose-response relationship of phototherapy for seasonal affective disorder: a meta-analysis. *Acta Psychiatr Scand* 1999; **99**:315–323.

Lewy AJ, Bauer VK, Cutler NL, Sack RL, Ahmed S, Thomas KH, Blood ML, Jackson JM. Morning vs evening light treatment of patients with winter depression. *Arch Gen Psychiatry* 1998; **55**:890–896.

Terman M, Terman JS, Quitkin FM, McGrath PJ, Stewart JW, Rafferty B. Light therapy for seasonal affective disorder. A review of efficacy. *Neuropsychopharmacology* 1989; **2**:1–22.

Terman M, Terman JS, Ross DC. A controlled trial of timed bright light and negative air ionization for treatment of winter depression. *Arch Gen Psychiatry* 1998; **55**:875–882.

Thompson C. Evidence-based treatment. In Partonen T, Magnusson A (eds). *Seasonal Affective Disorder: Practice and Research*. New York: Oxford University Press, 2001, pp. 151–158.

Wileman SM, Eagles JM, Andrew JE, Howie FL, Cameron IM, McCormack K, Naji SA. Light therapy for seasonal affective disorder in primary care: randomised controlled trial. *Br J Psychiatry* 2001; **178**:311–6.

Mechanism of action

Desan PH, Oren DA. Is seasonal affective disorder a disorder of circadian rhythms? *CNS Spectr* 2001; **6**:487–494.

Lam RW, Levitan RD. Pathophysiology of seasonal affective disorder: a review. *J Psychiatry Neurosci* 2000; **25**:469–480.

Lam RW, Tam EM, Yatham LN, Shiah IS, Zis AP. Seasonal depression: the dual vulnerability hypothesis revisited. *J Affect Disord* 2001; **63**:123–132.

Lewy AJ, Lefler BJ, Emens JS, Bauer VK. The circadian basis of winter depression. *Proc Natl Acad Sci USA* 2006; **103**:7414–7419.

McClung CA. Circadian genes, rhythms, and the biology of mood disorders. *Pharmacol Ther* 2007; **114**:222–232.

Sohn CH, Lam RW. Update on the biology of seasonal affective disorder. *CNS Spectr* 2005; **10**:635–646.

Wright HR, Lack LC, Kennaway DJ. Differential effects of light wavelength in phase advancing the melatonin rhythm. *J Pineal Res* 2004; **36**:140–144.

Young MA, Watel LG, Lahmeyer HW, Eastman CI. The temporal onset of individual symptoms in winter depression: differentiating underlying mechanisms. *J Affect Disord* 1991; **22**:191–197.

6

Light Treatment for Other Conditions

Although light therapy is widely associated with SAD, it is also being studied and used clinically in other conditions ranging from nonseasonal depression to bulimia nervosa to attention deficit hyperactivity disorder. This chapter will briefly review the evidence for therapeutic effects of light in these conditions and how we modify the light therapy method.

Nonseasonal depression

What's the evidence?

Nonseasonal depression is much more common than SAD so it is very important to determine whether light therapy might be effective for other types of MDD. There is some evidence for disrupted circadian rhythms in nonseasonal MDD, and light therapy may also have serotonergic and catecholaminergic effects, so there are certainly some plausible mechanisms for the beneficial effects of light.

However, despite the fact that light treatment was actually first investigated in nonseasonal depression (Kripke, 1981), fewer studies have been conducted of light therapy in nonseasonal MDD. Three systematic reviews of light therapy for nonseasonal MDD have shown some support for efficacy, but these are based on a small number of RCTs with methodological limitations, including small samples, short duration of treatment (averaging 7 days when light therapy was used alone), and inadequate placebo control conditions.

More recent, better-quality studies have investigated the use of bright light used in combination with antidepressants, with very promising results. For example, one well-designed trial conducted by Dr Klaus Martiny and colleagues in Denmark studied 102 patients with nonseasonal MDD, all started on the SSRI sertraline (Martiny, 2004). Patients were then randomized to sertraline (50 mg/d) combined with bright white light (10,000 lux fluorescent light for 60 minutes daily) or to sertraline combined with placebo dim red light (50 lux for 30 minutes daily) for 5 weeks; light treatments were all administered in the early morning.

They found significant benefit for sertraline combined with the active bright light on both clinician- and patient-rated scales. The percentage of responders (people with more than 50% improvement in depression scores) with the combined bright light and medication treatment was 67%, compared with 41% for the medication and placebo light. The differences were even more impressive for remission rate (percentage of the sample whose scores were in the normal range at study end): 42% for bright light combined with sertraline, vs. 15% for sertraline with placebo dim light. This study demonstrates that combined light and antidepressant treatment in nonseasonal MDD results in a clinically meaningful difference in response versus using an antidepressant alone.

In summary, although the evidence is still limited, there is a strong suggestion that light therapy is beneficial in nonseasonal unipolar depression. Given the mild side effects of light therapy, and the fact that light can be combined with other medications without worrying about drug–drug interactions, some investigators have recommended wider use of light therapy as an adjunctive treatment for nonseasonal MDD.

Practical aspects

The use of light therapy for mild to moderate nonseasonal MDD may be considered when the patient prefers a non-pharmacological treatment, or in combination with other treatments such as psychotherapy or pharmacotherapy. The light therapy method is the same as that used for SAD, with early morning light recommended.

Bipolar disorder

What's the evidence?

Bipolar disorder is another condition where light therapy may have great potential. There is increasing evidence for dysfunction of circadian rhythms in people with bipolar disorder, there are few validated treatments for the depressive phase of bipolar disorder, and often patients are on multiple medications so non-pharmacological treatments would be welcome.

SAD can be a bipolar condition as well, and many studies of light therapy in SAD have included some patients with bipolar disorder. In fact, Herb Kern, the first SAD patient to receive light therapy, had a bipolar disorder. Most of the studies, however, involve drug-free patients, so patients with bipolar II (with hypomanic episodes) disorder are more likely to be included than those with bipolar I (with manic episodes) disorder. While there are no published controlled studies directly comparing light therapy in unipolar and bipolar SAD, our clinical experience is that bipolar SAD patients also respond well to light.

In nonseasonal bipolar disorder, there is less clinical information about the effects of light and only small-sample pilot studies of light therapy. Light therapy has been used to treat subsyndromal winter depressive symptoms and also for rapid-cycling bipolar disorder, in which patients experience at least four mood episodes per year. A recent pilot study carefully examined the use of light therapy in nine women with bipolar depression (seven with bipolar I disorder and two with bipolar II disorder) (Sit et al., 2007). In that study, morning light exposure induced mixed mood states in three of the first four patients treated, so midday timing was used for the rest. The optimum response occurred with 7,000 lux given for 45–60 minutes at midday. Four of the nine patients had a sustained response to light therapy, either with midday or morning exposure, while two others had partial responses.

Another interesting use of bright light therapy being explored in bipolar disorder is to stabilize the usually transient effect of total sleep deprivation, now known as wake therapy. When depressed patients are kept awake all night, they often show an improvement in mood that continues through the next day. The mood changes can be dramatic, and many patients feel that their mood returns to baseline. Unfortunately, the mood improvement after sleep deprivation is not sustained. Most patients relapse after a recovery sleep the next day after sleep deprivation, and relapse can occur even after brief naps. However, the use of bright light after sleep deprivation may help to prevent these relapses. This may be particularly useful in bipolar disorder because antidepressants are not particularly effective and may worsen the clinical course. Dr Francesco Benedetti and Dr Anna Wirz-Justice have pioneered the use of this combination treatment in bipolar disorder (Benedetti et al., 2007). In collaboration with Dr Michael Terman, they have published a treatment manual for combining wake and light therapy (Wirz-Justice et al., 2009).

Practical aspects

Like other effective antidepressant treatments, light therapy can precipitate hypomanic or manic responses in susceptible patients, such as those with bipolar disorder. There has also been some suggestion that people with bipolar disorder are more biologically sensitive to light than normal subjects or those with unipolar depression. The immediate, energizing effect of bright light exposure can be experienced as agitation or feeling "revved up". Morning light exposure may exacerbate these effects. However, these effects usually subside rapidly when the light is stopped.

In our experience, patients with bipolar I disorder (with previous manic episodes) are more likely to experience agitation with light therapy and usually require dosage adjustment (e.g., reducing the time spent under the lights or sitting farther away from the light source). These patients should start with midday light exposure. If not optimally effective, and if agitation is not a problem, then they can be switched to morning timing. We also recommend that patients with bipolar I disorder be on a mood stabilizer medication when treated with light therapy.

Patients with bipolar II disorder (with hypomanic episodes) may not need a mood stabilizer medication if their hypomanic episodes are mild and infrequent. They can be treated with the morning light method as used for SAD. However, all patients with bipolar disorder should be cautioned about the risk of agitation, hypomania, and mixed states with bright light.

Medications used to treat bipolar disorder may also require special attention when prescribing light therapy (see Chapter 2). Lithium can affect the retina, although clinical studies of long-term lithium use have not shown any adverse retinal effects by clinical examination or by electrophysiological tests of retinal function. However, data from animal studies suggest that bright light exposure may potentiate some of the lithium-induced retinal changes. Similarly, other drugs such as phenothiazine antipsychotics (e.g., thioridazine) may potentially have photosensitizing effects. Ophthalmological consultation prior to light therapy and regular monitoring (e.g., annually) are recommended for patients taking these medications.

> **Clinical example**
>
> Sandra is diagnosed with bipolar II disorder with a seasonal pattern. She gets clinically depressed in the winter and mildly hypomanic in the summer. Lithium was introduced when she did not achieve full remission with light therapy during a winter depression. However, she did not like the side effects and so switched to lamotrigine. The medication, combined with light therapy, fully treats her winter depression.

Other depressive and psychiatric conditions

Depression during pregnancy and postpartum is very common and important to manage. When a mother is depressed, there are consequences for both her and her child. Non-pharmacological treatments are preferred because of the risk of drug effects on the fetus or the baby through breast milk. Light therapy would be an important addition to psychotherapies for these conditions. There are now preliminary studies showing that light may have beneficial effects during pregnancy. These are small studies and not well-controlled, so further evidence will need to be gathered before a general recommendation can be made.

Bulimia nervosa is an eating disorder that is characterized by binge-eating and purging by various means, including self-induced vomiting, laxative abuse, and excessive exercise. Over a dozen studies have shown that about 1/3 of women with bulimia have significant winter worsening of both mood and eating symptoms, and many also meet criteria for SAD. This may not be surprising, since serotonin is known to regulate appetite and may also be involved in the pathophysiology of both SAD and bulimia.

There have been several small placebo-controlled trials of light therapy for bulimia, with or without comorbid SAD. In all the studies there were significant therapeutic effects, either in reducing depressive symptoms, or in binge–purge frequency, or both. Given how difficult it is to treat bulimia, the use of light therapy can certainly be helpful especially when combined with standard treatments including cognitive behaviour therapy and antidepressant medications.

The menstrual cycle is an example of a biological rhythm that may also be influenced by the biological clock. Several studies have shown disturbances of circadian rhythms in women with premenstrual dysphoric disorder (PMDD, known colloquially as premenstrual syndrome, PMS, and in previous psychiatric terminology as late luteal phase dysphoric disorder, LLPDD). PMDD is also associated with SAD. One study found that 1/3 of women attending a PMS clinic had seasonality scores in the SAD range, indicating winter worsening of their PMS symptoms. Another study found that 46% of a group of women with SAD also had PMDD. A systematic review analysed four controlled trials of light therapy for PMDD (Krasnik et al., 2005). The overall conclusion was that there was a benefit of bright light but, because the studies had small samples, further evidence was required before "enthusiastic dissemination" could occur.

Recent research has also highlighted an association of attention deficit hyperactivity disorder (ADHD) with circadian dysfunction. For example, sleep complaints similar to delayed sleep phase syndrome (DSPS) are commonly seen in ADHD. We also know that bright light has alerting effects on concentration, so light therapy may also be of interest in this condition. Preliminary studies have indicated that light may have positive effects, so larger studies are currently under way.

Practical aspects

Given the evidence, even if preliminary, for beneficial effects of bright light in these conditions, it seems reasonable to offer light therapy as an adjunct to other treatments. The method for light therapy for bulimia, PMDD and ADHD is the same as that for SAD. While both morning and evening light exposure has been used in studies, we recommend starting with morning light, especially if there is winter worsening of symptoms. If there is little response, then a switch to evening light exposure can be tried.

Circadian sleep–wake disorders

There are many established disorders of circadian rhythms and sleep–wake timing, including circadian sleep disorders (DSPS, advanced sleep phase disorder, non-24 hour sleep–wake disorder), jet lag and shift work. The most common circadian sleep disorder is DSPS, otherwise known as the "night owl" syndrome. People with DSPS have a circadian clock that compels them to stay up late and sleep into the late morning, so their natural sleep time may be from 2:00 a.m. (or later) with natural waking time at 10:00 a.m. (or later). This is obviously a major problem if they need to function during regular work hours. This DSPS sleep–wake pattern is similar to that seen in people with SAD and in other disorders such as ADHD. DSPS is also found as a normal and transient developmental phase in adolescents and young adults.

Other circadian sleep disorders result from shift work and jet lag. In these conditions, the external environment changes in relation to internal clock time. Shift workers in particular have many disturbances in sleep, with resulting adverse effects on their health, including increased risk of accidents, cardiovascular disease, obesity, and cancer. The problem with shift workers is that their schedules and light exposure may be constantly changing. In addition, they often revert to a "normal" sleep–wake schedule on days off in order to interact with their families and friends. Thus, it is very difficult for them to synchronize their internal clocks with their external environments and they may be constantly "out of phase".

Age-related insomnia, which is often associated with an advanced sleep phase pattern (falling asleep early in the evening and waking up early in the morning), is a common problem for many older people. Circadian rhythm dysfunction is also implicated in behavioural disturbances in dementia, including the "sundowning" phenomenon. Several studies have shown beneficial effects of light therapy and increasing environmental light (to provide a stronger light–dark signal) in nursing homes. Recent studies have also found that bright room light in combination with melatonin may improve both cognitive and non-cognitive symptoms (including depression) in people with dementia.

Practical aspects

For DSPS, morning timing of light is indicated, as per the method for SAD. The use of the MEQ to select the optimal starting time for light therapy may also be helpful (see Chapter 2). Treatment for DSPS also includes avoidance of light in the evening. Conversely, advanced sleep phase disorder should be treated with evening bright light exposure and avoidance of light in the early morning. Light therapy may not be feasible for elderly people and nursing home residents because they have difficulty tolerating the bright light, but increasing the daytime environmental and room lighting may also be helpful.

It is very complicated to time light appropriately for other circadian sleep–wake disorders because the magnitude and direction of light-induced phase shifts is dependent on the timing of light exposure relative to the individual's circadian cycle (see Chapter 5). For these conditions, the timing of light depends on the starting circadian phase, the target circadian phase, and the length of time available for resynchronization. Jet lag calculators are available on the Internet to recommend the appropriate times for light exposure (and times to avoid bright light) based on your starting circadian phase, the direction of travel, and the number of time zones crossed, in order to optimize resynchronization of rhythms. Shift work optimization is best determined by experts associated with sleep disorders clinics.

Further reading

Benedetti F, Barbini B, Colombo C, Smeraldi E. Chronotherapeutics in psychiatric ward. *Sleep Med Rev* 2007; **11**:509–522.

Epperson CN, Terman M, Terman JS, Hanusa BH, Oren DA, Peindl KS, Wisner KL. Randomized clinical trial of bright light therapy for antepartum depression: preliminary findings. *J Clin Psychiatry* 2004; **65**:421–425.

Even C, Schroder CM, Friedman S, Rouillon F. Efficacy of light therapy in nonseasonal depression: a systematic review. *J Affect Disord* 2008; **108**:11–23.

Fahey CD, Zee PC. Circadian rhythm sleep disorders and phototherapy. *Psychiatr Clin North Am* 2006; **29**:989–1007.

Gammack JK. Light therapy for insomnia in older adults. *Clin Geriatr Med* 2008 Feb; **24**(1):139–149.

Lam RW (ed). *Seasonal Affective Disorder and Beyond: Light Treatment for SAD and non-SAD Conditions.* Washington, DC: American Psychiatric Press, 1998.

Krasnik C, Montori VM, Guyatt GH, Heels-Ansdell D, Busse JW. Medically Unexplained Syndromes Study Group. The effect of bright light therapy on depression associated with premenstrual dysphoric disorder. *Am J Obstet Gynecol* 2005; **193**:658–661.

Kripke DF. Photoperiodic mechanisms for depression and its treatment. In Perris C, Struwe G, Janson B (eds). *Biological Psychiatry.* Amsterdam: Elsevier, 1981.

Martiny K. Adjunctive bright light in nonseasonal major depression. *Acta Psychiatr Scand Suppl* 2004; 7–28.

Riemersma-van der Lek RF, Swaab DF, Twisk J, Hol EM, Hoogendijk WJ, Van Someren EJ. Effect of bright light and melatonin on cognitive and noncognitive function in elderly residents of group care facilities: a randomized controlled trial. *JAMA* 2008; **299**:2642–2655.

Sit D, Wisner KL, Hanusa BH, Stull S, Terman M. Light therapy for bipolar disorder: a case series in women. *Bipolar Disord* 2007; **9**:918–927.

Terman M, Terman JS. Light therapy for seasonal and nonseasonal depression: efficacy, protocol, safety, and side effects. *CNS Spectr* 2005; **10**:647–663.

Terman M, Terman JS. Light therapy. In Kryger MH, Roth T, Dement WC (eds). *Principles and Practice of Sleep Medicine.* 4th edition. Philadelphia: Elsevier, 2005, pp. 1424–1442.

Terman M. Evolving applications of light therapy. *Sleep Med Rev* 2007; **11**:497–507.

Tuunainen A, Kripke DF, Endo T. Light therapy for nonseasonal depression. *Cochrane Database Syst Rev* 2004; CD004050.

Wirz-Justice A, Benedetti F, Terman M. *Chronotherapeutics for Affective Disorders.* Basel: Karger, 2009.

7

Clinician Resources

- Internet and print resources
- Audit Form – chart review
- Frequently Asked Questions (FAQs) about SAD
- Instructions for Light Therapy handout
- Patient Self-Care handout
- MEQ
- SPAQ
- SIGH-SAD Summary
- PHQ-9
- QIDS-SR
- Adverse Events Scale
- Sample insurance reimbursement letter

Internet and print resources

Useful Internet sites

www. UBCsad.ca	SAD Information Page at the University of BC . Our site includes many of the resources in this chapter, available for free download.
www.sltbr.org	Society for Light Treatment and Biological Rhythms (SLTBR). SLTBR is an international, not-for-profit society dedicated to fostering research, professional development and clinical applications in the fields of light therapy and biological rhythms. The site includes a list of Corporate Members that manufacture and distribute light devices.
www.cet.org	Center for Environmental Therapeutics. This site includes information on recent research and treatment, on-line screening and assessment tools for the public, and a clinician assessment package to order.
www.sada. org.uk	The Seasonal Affective Disorder Association Based in the UK, this is the world's longest-established support organization for those with SAD. The site includes a low-cost information pack available to order.

Books for clinicians and researchers

Seasonal Affective Disorder and Beyond. Light Treatment for SAD and Non-SAD Conditions. Raymond W. Lam (editor), American Psychiatric Press Inc., 1998.

Canadian Consensus Guidelines for the Treatment of Seasonal Affective Disorder. Raymond W. Lam, Anthony J. Levitt (editors), Clinical and Academic Publishing, 1999. Available for free download at www.UBCsad.ca

Seasonal Affective Disorder: Practice and Research. Second Edition. Timo Partonen, Andres Magnusson (editors), Oxford University Press, 2009.

Coping with the Seasons. A Cognitive Behavioral Approach for Seasonal Affective Disorder. Therapist Guide. Kelly J. Rohan, Oxford University Press, 2008.

Chronotherapeutics for Affective Disorders. Anna Wirz-Justice, Francesco Benedetti, Michael Terman, Karger Press, 2009.

Audit Form – chart review

This checklist helps you to audit your practice to ensure that you are meeting recommended clinical guidelines. Pull the charts of the last 10 patients whom you have seen in the past 12 months for whom you have made the diagnosis of depressive disorder or SAD, and review whether the recommendations have been followed.

Clinician behaviour	Yes	No
Diagnosis		
• Checked for atypical features?		
• Checked for recurrent seasonal episodes?		
• Checked for summer remissions?		
• Checked for regular seasonal psychosocial stressors?		
• Checked for eating disorders?		
• Checked for summer hypomania/mania?		
• Checked for winter worsening of depression?		
• Checked relevant laboratory tests, e.g., TSH?		
Management – Light Therapy		
• Discussed light therapy?		
• Warned against suntan studio use?		
• Checked for retinal and systemic risk factors?		
• Advised light therapy with 10,000 lux light box?		
• Checked specifications of light box used?		
• Discussed reimbursement issues re: light boxes?		
• Advised light therapy for at least 30 minutes per day?		
• Advised light therapy in early morning?		
• Advised light therapy daily for at least 2 weeks?		

• Checked for side effects to light therapy?		
• Checked response to light therapy?		
• Used a rating scale to check response?		
• Advised when to stop light therapy in the spring?		
• Advised when to restart light therapy next season?		
Management – Antidepressants		
• Checked whether antidepressant medication needed?		
• Used an SSRI (fluoxetine, sertraline) or bupropion as first-line medication?		
• Checked side effects/response to antidepressant?		
• Advised when to stop antidepressant?		
Management – Combined Light Therapy/Antidepressant		
• Considered monotherapy before combination therapy?		
• Used combined light therapy/antidepressant?		
• Checked side effects/response to light therapy/antidepressant?		

Frequently Asked Questions (FAQ) about SAD

This is a helpful educational brochure about SAD for patients, family, friends and the public.

Frequently Asked Questions about Seasonal Affective Disorder (SAD)

What is SAD? How is it different from the winter blues?

Many people feel mildly "depressed" during the winter, but some people have more severe bouts of feeling down all the time, low energy, problems with sleep and appetite, loss of interest, and reduced concentration to the point where they have difficulty functioning at work or in the home. We say that these people have a clinical depression, to distinguish it from everyday ups and downs. Seasonal affective disorder ("affective" is a psychiatric term for mood), or SAD, describes people who have these clinical depressions only during the autumn and winter seasons. During the spring and summer, they feel well and "normal".

Other common symptoms of SAD include oversleeping, extreme fatigue, increased appetite with carbohydrate craving, overeating, and weight gain. With more severe episodes, people may have suicidal thoughts.

How common is SAD?

Researchers believe that SAD results from the shorter day length in winter. Recent studies estimate that SAD is more common in northern countries because the winter day gets shorter as you go farther north. Studies in Ontario suggest that 1% to 3% of the general population have SAD. This means that up to 1 million in Canada may have difficulties in the winter due to significant clinical depression. Another 15% of people have the "winter blues" or "winter blahs" – winter symptoms similar to SAD, but not to the point of having a clinical depression.

What treatments are available for SAD?

Research has shown that many patients with SAD improve with exposure to bright, artificial light, called light therapy, or phototherapy. As little as 30 minutes per day of sitting under a specially designed light device results in significant improvement in 60% to 70% of patients with SAD.

How do you use light therapy?

A fluorescent light box is the best-studied light therapy treatment. People usually purchase a light box and use it in their own homes. The usual "dose" of light is 10,000 lux, where lux is a measurement of light intensity. Indoor light is usually less than 400 lux; a cloudy day about 3,000 lux; and a sunny day is 50,000 lux or more. Using the 10,000 lux light box for about 30 minutes a day is usually enough for a beneficial response. A light box with a lower lux rating usually requires more time for a response. For example, 5,000 lux light boxes usually require 45–60 minutes of daily exposure, while 2,500 lux light boxes require 1–2 hours of exposure.

Other light devices are also commercially available. Some devices use light-emitting diodes (LEDs) which are longer-lasting and are much smaller and more portable than light boxes. Light visors and other head-mounted units can offer more portability than light boxes. Dawn simulators are devices that gradually increase the lights in the bedroom to "simulate" a summer dawn in the winter. While these devices can be beneficial for some people, there is less evidence to show that they are effective for SAD compared to light boxes.

Most light devices use white light. Currently, blue-light devices are NOT recommended because they have not been extensively tested, there is no indication that blue light is better than white light for SAD, and there is no information on long-term safety (unlike white-light devices). There are some theoretical reasons why blue light may be harmful to the eyes.

What about sun tanning studios?

People are cautioned NOT to use sun tanning studios to treat SAD because there is NO evidence that they are helpful. The effect of light therapy is through the eyes, not through skin exposure, and people should not open their eyes in tanning booths because of the harmful effects of ultraviolet exposure. Fluorescent light boxes have filters to block the harmful ultraviolet rays and LED lights do not emit ultraviolet wavelengths.

How do I get a light box?

Safe and portable light devices are now commercially available.
Ask your doctor, or contact our clinic for more information (or check
our web site at www.UBCsad.ca). The cost of a light box is usually between
$150 and $300 (Canadian). We do not recommend building your own light
box, because of the safety hazards, and the difficulty in getting the correct
dose of light.

Are there side effects to light therapy?

Side effects of light therapy are usually mild. Some people may experience
mild nausea, headaches, eyestrain, or feeling "edgy" when they first start
using light therapy. These effects usually get better with time or reducing the
light exposure. People who have bipolar disorder (manic-depressive illness)
should consult their doctor before using light therapy.

There are no known long-term harmful effects of light therapy.
However, people with certain medical conditions (such as retinal disease,
macular degeneration or diabetes) or taking certain medications (such as
thioridazine, lithium or melatonin) should have special eye examinations
before considering light therapy.

Are there other treatments for SAD?

Other treatments for depression, including the newer antidepressant
medications (e.g., selective serotonin reuptake inhibitors, or SSRIs such as
fluoxetine [Prozac]; bupropion-XL [Wellbutrin]; moclobemide [Manerix];
and others) are also effective for patients with SAD and can be used to
prevent episodes. Counselling or cognitive-behaviour therapy may also help.
People with milder symptoms of the "winter blues" may be helped by simply
spending more time outdoors and exercising regularly in the winter (e.g., a
daily noon-hour walk).

Some people with SAD find that they also feel better by increasing the
indoor light in their homes and/or offices, painting their walls in light

colours, and sitting near windows for natural light. There is no evidence, however, that these activities alone can treat SAD.

What causes SAD and how does light therapy work?

We don't know, exactly, but research shows that light has a biological effect on brain chemicals (neurotransmitters) and function. One theory is that people with SAD have a disturbance in the "biological clock" in the brain that regulates hormones, sleep and mood, so that this clock "runs slow" in the winter. The bright light may help to "reset the clock" and restore normal function. Other theories are that neurotransmitter functions, particularly serotonin and dopamine, are disturbed in SAD, and that these neurotransmitter imbalances are corrected by light therapy and/or antidepressant medications. Still other scientists believe that patients with SAD have reduced retinal light sensitivity or immune function in the winter that is corrected by light therapy. There is also evidence for a genetic contribution to SAD.

What should I do if I think I have SAD?

Everyone who is significantly depressed should be assessed by their family doctor because some physical problems (e.g., thyroid disease) can show up as depression. People with SAD can be treated by their family doctor or referred to a psychiatrist, psychologist or other health professional who is knowledgeable about SAD. To find a SAD specialist, check with the nearest university medical school department of psychiatry. People should not treat themselves with light exposure until after assessment by a qualified health professional.

Can I read more about SAD?

Check our website at www.UBCsad.ca, or this book:

Winter Blues: Everything you Need to Know to Beat Seasonal Affective Disorder, by Dr. Norman Rosenthal (one of the pioneer researchers in SAD and light therapy). Guilford Press, revised 2005, about $18.00 (Cdn).

Instructions for Light Therapy handout

Instructions for using Light Therapy

Note that this information does not substitute for medical consultation. You should always check out information with your own doctor. These instructions should ONLY be used in conjunction with supervision by a qualified health professional.

1 These instructions are for fluorescent light boxes that emit 10,000 lux light (lux is a measurement of light intensity). Light boxes with lower lux rating usually require more time for response. For example, 5,000 lux light boxes usually require 45–60 minutes of daily exposure, while 2,500 lux light boxes require 1–2 hours of exposure.

2 Other light devices are also commercially available (e.g., LED lights, light visors, dawn simulators). They may be beneficial for some patients, but there is less evidence to show that they are effective compared to light boxes. When using these devices, follow the instructions from the manufacturer.

3 The light boxes we recommend contain cool-white fluorescent lights, but full-spectrum fluorescent lights are also effective (although more expensive). The light box should have an ultraviolet filter.
Do not use sunlamps, tanning lamps or halogen lamps as these may be harmful to your eyes!

4 During light therapy, you should keep to a regular sleep schedule (going to sleep and waking up at regular times, for example, 11:00 p.m. to 7:00 a.m.).

5 The light box should be placed on a table or counter so that you can sit comfortably. You must be positioned correctly, so follow the manufacturer's information about the distance to the light box.

6 You can read or eat while sitting under the lights, but your eyes must be open for the effect to occur. You cannot sleep during your light exposure! You should **not** stare directly at the lights.

7 Start with 30 minutes of light exposure per day. Start light therapy in the early morning, as soon as possible after awakening (between 6:00 a.m. and 9:00 a.m.).

8   Response usually starts in a few days, and by two weeks the symptoms should be definitely improving. Most people need to continue light therapy throughout the winter until the springtime. When light therapy is stopped, symptoms do not usually reappear for a few days, so most people can stop the treatment for one or two days without much problem (e.g., for a weekend trip).

9   If the symptoms are **NOT** improving after 14 days, try spending up to 60 minutes per day in front of lights each morning, or divided between the morning and evening. Do not use the light box too near bedtime, as the light exposure can disturb sleep. If this still does not help, contact your doctor.

10 When there is a good response to light therapy, some patients like to experiment with the timing and duration of daily light exposure, e.g., by reducing the daily exposure to 15 minutes, or using the light at a more convenient time of the day (e.g., 7:00 p.m.). We suggest making one change at a time, for 2 weeks. If symptoms start returning, go back to the original dosing schedule.

11 There are no reported harmful effects on the eyes with light therapy as described, but the long-term effects have not yet been studied. If you have eye problems (e.g., retinal disease, macular degeneration, or diabetes), or worries about eye damage, please tell your doctor.

12 Some people experience mild headaches, nausea, dizziness or eye strain when using the lights. These symptoms usually occur at the beginning of treatment, and get better in a few days. Otherwise, they can be relieved by reducing the daily exposure time, or by sitting slightly farther away from the lights.

13 Occasionally people report feeling irritable, or euphoric, or being "too high" when treated with light therapy. If this happens, the treatment should be stopped, and you should contact your doctor. If light therapy is restarted, use a shorter exposure time (e.g., 15 minutes per day) or sit slightly farther away from the lights. People with bipolar disorder (manic-depressive illness) should consult with their doctor before using light therapy.

Patient Self-Care handout

Self-Care Tips for Winter Blues and Seasonal Affective Disorder (SAD)

- Educate your self, family and close friends about SAD to gain their understanding and support. Here are some helpful web sites for more information and support:
  - ➢ SAD Information Page at the University of BC. Our site includes many resources available for free download. www.UBCsad.ca
  - ➢ Center for Environmental Therapeutics. Includes information on recent research and treatment, on-line screening and assessment tools for the public. www.cet.org
  - ➢ The Seasonal Affective Disorder Association. Based in the UK, this is the world's longest-established support organization for those with SAD. The site includes a low-cost information pack available to order. www.sada.org.uk
- Share experiences regarding SAD and treatment with others for information, understanding, validation and support. Here are some helpful books on the topic:
  - ➢ *Winter Blues, Revised Edition. Everything You Need to Know to Beat Seasonal Affective Disorder*. By Norman E. Rosenthal, Guilford Press, 2006, about $28.
  - ➢ *Coping with the Seasons. A Cognitive Behavioral Approach for Seasonal Affective Disorder. Workbook*. By Kelly J. Rohan, Oxford University Press, 2008, about $30.
  - ➢ *Seasonal Affective Disorder for Dummies*. By Laura L. Smith and Charles H. Elliott, Wiley Press, 2007, about $22.
- Get as much light as possible and avoid dark environments during daylight hours in winter.
- Rearrange workspaces at home and work near a window, or set up bright lights in your work area. Allow natural light to shine through open windows when temperatures are moderate.
- Consider going without sunglasses in the winter except in very bright sun/snow or decrease the amount of time wearing them.
- Be aware of cold outdoor temperatures and dress to conserve energy and warmth. Many affected by seasonal changes report sensitivity to extreme temperatures.
- Reduce mild winter depressive symptoms by exercising daily – outdoors when possible to take advantage of natural light, but inside is okay too.

- Stay on a regular sleep/wake schedule. People who get up every morning and go to sleep at the same time report being more alert and less fatigued than when they vary their schedules.
- Try putting your bedroom lights on a timer set to switch on ½ hour or more before awakening. Some people report it is easier to wake up when using this technique with lights.
- Some find it helpful to record their biological rhythms during fall and winter. Try keeping a daily log noting weather conditions and your energy levels, moods, appetite/weight, sleep times and activities.
- Arrange family outings and social occasions for day times and early evening in winter. Avoid staying up late, which disrupts the sleep schedule and biological clock.
- Postpone making major life changes until spring or summer when possible.
- If you are able, arrange a winter vacation to a warm, sunny climate!

Morningness-Eveningness Questionnaire (MEQ)

- The MEQ is a questionnaire developed by Horne and Ostberg based on the concept of chronotype, or the degree to which one is a morning person (a lark) or an evening person (an owl).
- The MEQ score has also been correlated with circadian phase and has been used to predict the timing of light therapy. The scoring of the MEQ can be categorized as:

MEQ Score	Morningness-Eveningness
16–30	Definite evening type
31–41	Moderate evening type
42–58	Intermediate (neither morning nor evening type)
59–69	Moderate morning type
70–86	Definite morning type

Horne JA, Ostberg O. A self-assessment questionnaire to determine morningness-eveningness in human circadian rhythms. *Int J Chronobiol* 1976; 4:97–110.

Morningness-Eveningness Questionnaire (MEQ)

Instructions:

- Please read each question very carefully before answering.
- Please answer each question as honestly as possible.
- Answer ALL questions.
- Each question should be answered independently of others. Do NOT go back and check your answers.

1. What time would you get up if you were entirely free to plan your day?

5:00 – 6:30 a.m.	5
6:30 – 7:45 a.m.	4
7:45 – 9:45 a.m.	3
9:45 – 11:00 a.m.	2
11:00 a.m. – 12 Noon	1
12 Noon – 5:00 a.m.	0

2. What time would you go to bed if you were entirely free to plan your evening?

8:00 – 9:00 p.m.	5
9:00 – 10:15 p.m.	4
10:15 p.m. – 12:30 a.m.	3
12:30 – 1:45 a.m.	2
1:45 – 3:00 a.m.	1
3:00 a.m. – 8:00 p.m.	0

3. If there is a specific time at which you have to get up in the morning, to what extent do you depend on being woken up by an alarm clock?

Not at all dependent	4
Slightly dependent	3
Fairly dependent	2
Very dependent	1

4. **How easy do you find it to get up in the morning (when you are not woken up unexpectedly)?**

Not at all easy	1
Not very easy	2
Fairly easy	3
Very easy	4

5. **How alert do you feel during the first half-hour after you wake up in the morning?**

Not at all alert	1
Slightly alert	2
Fairly alert	3
Very alert	4

6. **How hungry do you feel during the first half-hour after you wake up in the morning?**

Not at all hungry	1
Slightly hungry	2
Fairly hungry	3
Very hungry	4

7. **During the first half-hour after you wake up in the morning, how tired do you feel?**

Very tired	1
Fairly tired	2
Fairly refreshed	3
Very refreshed	4

8. **If you have no commitments the next day, what time would you go to bed compared to your usual bedtime?**

Seldom or never later	4
Less than one hour later	3
1–2 hours later	2
More than two hours later	1

9. **You have decided to engage in some physical exercise. A friend suggests that you do this for one hour twice a week, and the best time for him is between 7:00 and 8:00 a.m. Bearing in mind nothing but your own internal "clock", how do you think you would perform?**

Would be in good form	4
Would be in reasonable form	3
Would find it difficult	2
Would find it very difficult	1

10. **At what time of day do you feel you become tired as a result of need for sleep?**

8:00 – 9:00 p.m.	5
9:00 – 10:15 p.m.	4
10:15 p.m. – 12:45 a.m.	3
12:45 – 2:00 a.m.	2
2:00 – 3:00 a.m.	1

11. **You want to be at your peak performance for a test that you know is going to be mentally exhausting and will last for two hours. You are entirely free to plan your day. Considering only your own internal "clock", which ONE of the four testing times would you choose?**

8:00 – 10:00 a.m.	4
11:00 a.m. – 1:00 p.m.	3
3:00 – 5:00 p.m.	2
7:00 – 9:00 p.m.	1

12. **If you got into bed at 11:00 p.m., how tired would you be?**

Not at all tired	1
A little tired	2
Fairly tired	3
Very tired	4

13. **For some reason you have gone to bed several hours later than usual, but there is no need to get up at any particular time the next morning. Which ONE of the following are you most likely to do?**

Will wake up at usual time, but will NOT fall back asleep	4
Will wake up at usual time and will doze thereafter	3
Will wake up at usual time but will fall asleep again	2
Will NOT wake up until later than usual	1

14. **One night you have to remain awake between 4:00 and 6:00 a.m. in order to carry out a night watch. You have no commitments the next day. Which ONE of the alternatives will suit you best?**

Would NOT go to bed until watch was over	1
Would take a nap before and sleep after	2
Would take a good sleep before and nap after	3
Would sleep only before watch	4

15. **You have to do two hours of hard physical work. You are entirely free to plan your day. Considering only your own internal "clock", which ONE of the following times would you choose?**

8:00 – 10:00 a.m.	4
11:00 a.m. – 1:00 p.m.	3
3:00 – 5:00 p.m.	2
7:00 – 9:00 p.m.	1

16. **You have decided to engage in hard physical exercise. A friend suggests that you do this for one hour twice a week and the best time for him is between 10:00 and 11:00 p.m. Bearing in mind nothing else but your own internal "clock," how well do you think you would perform?**

Would be in good form	1
Would be in reasonable form	2
Would find it difficult	3
Would find it very difficult	4

17. **Suppose that you can choose your own work hours. Assume that you worked a FIVE hour day (including breaks) and that your job was interesting and paid by results). Which FIVE CONSECUTIVE HOURS would you select?**

5 hours starting between 4:00 and 8:00 a.m.	5
5 hours starting between 8:00 and 9:00 a.m.	4
5 hours starting between 9:00 a.m. and 2:00 p.m.	3
5 hours starting between 2:00 and 5:00 p.m.	2
5 hours starting between 5:00 p.m. and 4:00 a.m.	1

18. **At what time of the day do you think that you reach your "feeling best" peak?**

5:00 – 8:00 a.m.	5
8:00 – 10:00 a.m.	4
10:00 a.m. – 5:00 p.m.	3
5:00 – 10:00 p.m.	2
10:00 p.m. – 5:00 a.m.	1

19. **One hears about "morning" and "evening" types of people. Which ONE of these types do you consider yourself to be?**

Definitely a "morning" type	6
Rather more a "morning" than an "evening" type	4
Rather more an "evening" than a "morning" type	2
Definitely an "evening" type	0

Seasonal Pattern Assessment Questionnaire (SPAQ)

- The SPAQ is a widely used screening questionnaire for seasonality.
- The Global Seasonality Score (GSS) is the total sum of the six items on Question 11. This gives a score from 0 (no seasonality) to 24 (extreme seasonality). The average GSS in community samples is about 5. The average GSS in patients with SAD is about 16.
- The screening criteria for a "diagnosis" of SAD are based on the GSS and the score on Question 17, the degree of problems associated with seasonal changes.
- A GSS of **11** or higher and a score on Q.11 of **moderate** or greater is indicative of SAD.
- As with most screening questionnaires, these criteria tend to overdiagnose SAD. On clinical interview, some people with these criteria will turn out to have subsyndromal features. On the other hand, very few people with a true diagnosis of SAD will be missed using these criteria.

Mersch PP, Vastenburg NC, Meesters Y, Bouhuys AL, Beersma DG, Van den Hoofdakker RH, den Boer JA. The reliability and validity of the Seasonal Pattern Assessment Questionnaire: a comparison between patient groups. *J Affect Disord* 2004; 80:209–219.

CHAPTER 7

SEASONAL PATTERN ASSESSMENT QUESTIONNAIRE (SPAQ)

1. Name _____   2. Age _____

3. Place of birth - City / Province (State) / Country _____

4. Today's date   _____   _____   _____
                        Month   Day   Year

5. Current weight (in lbs.) _____

6. Years of education   Less than four years of high school   1

                         High school only   2

                         1-3 years post high school   3

                         4 or more years post high school   4

7. Sex -   Male   1   Female   2

8. Marital Status -   Single   1
                       Married   2
                       Sep./Divorced   3
                       Widowed   4

9. Occupation   _____

10. How many years have you lived in this climatic area?   _____

> INSTRUCTIONS
>
> * Please circle the number beside your choice.
>
> Example:
> Sex Male [1]   Female 2

The purpose of this form is to find out how your mood and behaviour change over time. Please fill in all the relevant circles. Note: We are interested in your experience; <u>not others</u> you may have observed.

---

11. To what degree do the following change with the seasons?

	No Change	Slight Change	Moderate Change	Marked Change	Extremely Marked Change
A. Sleep length	0	1	2	3	4
B. Social activity	0	1	2	3	4
C. Mood (overall feeling of well-being)	0	1	2	3	4
D. Weight	0	1	2	3	4
E. Appetite	0	1	2	3	4
F. Energy level	0	1	2	3	4

12. In the following questions, fill in circles for all applicable months. This may be a single month O, a cluster of months, e.g. O O O , or any other grouping.

At what time of year do you....

	Jan	Feb	Mar	Apr	May	Jun	Jul	Aug	Sep	Oct	Nov	Dec	OR	No particular month(s) stand out as extreme on a regular basis
A. Feel best	O	O	O	O	O	O	O	O	O	O	O	O		O
B. Gain most weight	O	O	O	O	O	O	O	O	O	O	O	O		O
C. Socialize most	O	O	O	O	O	O	O	O	O	O	O	O		O
D. Sleep least	O	O	O	O	O	O	O	O	O	O	O	O		O
E. Eat most	O	O	O	O	O	O	O	O	O	O	O	O	OR	O
F. Lose most weight	O	O	O	O	O	O	O	O	O	O	O	O		O
G. Socialize least	O	O	O	O	O	O	O	O	O	O	O	O		O
H. Feel worst	O	O	O	O	O	O	O	O	O	O	O	O		O
I. Eat least	O	O	O	O	O	O	O	O	O	O	O	O		O
J. Sleep most	O	O	O	O	O	O	O	O	O	O	O	O		O

14. How much does your weight fluctuate during the course of the year?

0-3 lbs	1	12-15 lbs	4
4-7 lbs	2	16-20 lbs	5
8-11 lbs	3	Over 20 lbs	6

15. Approximately how many hours of each 24-hour day do you sleep during each season? (Include naps)

Winter	0 1 2 3 4 5 6 7 8 9 10 11 12 13 14 15 16 17 18 Over18
Spring	0 1 2 3 4 5 6 7 8 9 10 11 12 13 14 15 16 17 18 Over18
Summer	0 1 2 3 4 5 6 7 8 9 10 11 12 13 14 15 16 17 18 Over18
Fall	0 1 2 3 4 5 6 7 8 9 10 11 12 13 14 15 16 17 18 Over18

16. Do you notice a change in food preference during the different seasons?

No   1   Yes   2   If yes, please specify :

17. If you experience changes with the seasons, do you feel that these are a problems for you?

No   1   Yes   2   If yes, is this problem -   mild   1

moderate   2

marked   3

severe   4

disabling   5

Thank you for completing this questionnaire.

* Raymond W. Lam 1998 (modified from Rosenthal, Bradt and Wehr 1987).

Structured Interview Guide for the Hamilton Depression Rating Scale, SAD version (SIGH-SAD) Summary

- The Hamilton Depression Rating Scale (Ham-D) is the most widely used outcome scale for depression studies. The Ham-D is based on a clinical interview with the patient and is rated by the interviewer. The interviewer asks the patient about symptoms experienced in the past week, compared to a time when they were well. A structured interview guide is also available (Williams, 1988).
- There are various versions of the Ham-D, which was originally developed in the 1960s. The original version (17 items, Ham-17) and a later version (with an additional four items, Ham-21) did not include items rating atypical symptoms (such as oversleeping, overeating, weight gain, etc.). An 8-item atypical symptom addendum was added to rate these symptoms. The resulting 29-item version (Ham-29) is widely used in SAD studies.
- However, the four additional items (including the diurnal variation item) on the Ham-21 and one item on the Ham-8 are not related to severity of depression. Hence, the Ham-24 (sum of the Ham-17 and Ham-7) is a better indicator of severity than the Ham-29.
- The Ham-24 and Ham-29 scores can be categorized this way:

Category	Ham-24 score	Ham-29 score
Normal, not depressed	9 or less	11 or less
Mildly depressed	10 to 19	12 to 21
Moderately depressed	20 to 29	22 to 32
Markedly/severely depressed	30 or more	33 or more

Williams JB. A structured interview guide for the Hamilton Depression Rating Scale. *Arch Gen Psychiatry* 1988; 45:742–747.

SIGH-SAD (Ham-D) Summary Score Sheet

1. Depressed Mood

0 = Absent.
1 = These feeling states indicated only on questioning.
2 = These feeling states spontaneously reported verbally.
3 = Communicates feeling states non-verbally – i.e., through facial expression, posture, voice, and tendency to weep.
4 = Patient reports virtually only these feeling states in his spontaneous verbal and non-verbal communication.

2. Work and Activities

0 = No difficulty.
1 = Thoughts and feelings of incapacity, fatigue or weakness related to activities; work or hobbies.
2 = Loss of interest in activities; hobbies or work – either directly reported by patient, or indirect in listlessness, indecision and vacillation (feels he has to push self to work or activities).
3 = Decrease in actual time spent in activities or decrease in productivity. In hospital rate 3 if patient does not spend at least three hours a day in activities (hospital job or hobbies) exclusive of ward chores.
4 = Stopped working because of present illness. In hospital, rate 4 if patient engages in no activities except ward chores, or if patient fails to perform ward chores unassisted.

3. Social Withdrawal

0 = Interacts with other people as usual.
1 = Less interested in socializing with others but continues to do so.
2 = Interacting less with other people in social (optional) situations.
3 = Interacting less with other people in work or family situations (i.e. where this is necessary).
4 = Marked withdrawal from others in family or work situations.

4. Genital Symptoms

0 = Absent.
1 = Mild.
2 = Severe.

5. Somatic Symptoms – GI

0 = None.
1 = Loss of appetite but eating without staff encouragement. Heavy feelings in abdomen.
2 = Difficulty eating without staff urging. Requests or requires laxatives or medication for bowels or medication for GI symptoms.

6. Loss of Weight

0 = No weight loss.
1 = Probable weight loss associated with present illness.
2 = Definite (according to patient) weight loss.

7. Weight Gain

0 = No weight gain.
1 = Probable weight gain due to current depression.
2 = Definite (according to patient) weight gain due to depression.

8. Appetite Increase

0 = No increase in appetite.
1 = Wants to eat a little more than usual.
2 = Wants to eat somewhat more than normal.
3 = Wants to eat much more than usual.

9. Increased Eating

0 = Is not eating more than usual.
1 = Is eating a little more than usual.
2 = Is eating somewhat more than usual.
3 = Is eating much more than normal.

10. Carbohydrate Craving

0 = No change in food preference or consumption.
1 = Craving or eating more carbohydrates (starches or sugars) than before.
2 = Craving or eating much more carbohydrates than before.
3 = Irresistible craving or eating of sweets or starches.

11. Insomnia – Early

0 = No difficulty falling asleep.
1 = Complains of occasional difficulty falling asleep – i.e., more than 1/2 hour.
2 = Complains of nightly difficulty falling asleep.

12. Insomnia – Middle

0 = No difficulty.
1 = Patient complains of being restless and disturbed during the night.
2 = Waking during the night – any getting out of bed rates 2 (except for purposes of voiding).

13. Insomnia – late

0 = No difficulty.
1 = Waking in early hours of the morning but goes back to sleep.
2 = Unable to fall asleep again if patient gets out of bed.

14. Hypersomnia

0 = No increase in sleep length.
1 = At least 1 hour increase in sleep length.
2 = 2+ hour increase.
3 = 3+ hour increase.
4 = 4+ hour increase.

15. Somatic Symptoms – General

0 = None.
1 = Heaviness in limbs, back or head. Backaches, headache, muscle aches. Loss of energy and fatigability.
2 = Any clear-cut symptom rates 2.

16. Fatigability

0 = Does not feel more fatigued than usual.
1 = Feels more fatigued than usual but this has not impaired function significantly; less frequent than in (2).
2 = More fatigued than usual; at least one hour a day; at least three days a week.
3 = Fatigued much of the time most days.
4 = Fatigued almost all the time.

17. Feelings of Guilt

0 = Absent.
1 = Self reproach, feels he has let people down.
2 = Ideas of guilt or rumination over past errors or sinful deeds.

3 = Present illness is a punishment. Delusions of guilt.
4 = Hears accusatory or denunciatory voices and/or experiences threatening visual hallucinations.

18. Suicide

0 = Absent.
1 = Feels life is not worth living.
2 = Wishes he were dead or any thoughts of possible death to self.
3 = Suicide ideas or gestures.
4 = Attempts at suicide (any serious attempt rates 4).

19. Anxiety – Psychic

0 = No difficulty.
1 = Subjective tension and irritability.
2 = Worrying about minor matters.
3 = Apprehensive attitude apparent in face or speech.
4 = Fears expressed without questioning.

20. Anxiety – Somatic

0 = Absent.
1 = Mild.
2 = Moderate.
3 = Severe.
4 = Incapacitating.

21. Hypochondriasis

0 = Not present
1 = Self-absorption (bodily).
2 = Preoccupation with health.
3 = Frequent complaints, requests for help, etc.
4 = Hypochondriacal delusions.

22. Insight

0 = Acknowledges being depressed and ill.
1 = Acknowledges illness but attributes cause to bad food, climate, overwork, virus, need for rest, etc.
2 = Denies being ill at all.

23. Motor Retardation

0 = Normal speech and thought.
1 = Slight retardation at interview.
2 = Obvious retardation at interview.
3 = Interview difficult.
4 = Complete stupor.

24. Agitation

0 = None.
1 = Fidgetiness.
2 = Playing with hands, hair, etc.
3 = Moving about, can't sit still.
4 = Hand wringing, nail biting, hair pulling, biting of lips.

17-item Ham-D Total: _____
(do not include shaded items)

7-item Atypical Total: _____
(only shaded items)

24-item Ham-D Total: _____
(all items)

25. Diurnal Variation

0 = None.
1 = Mild.
　　Worse in:　a.m.　p.m.
2 = Severe.

26. Reverse Diurnal (Afternoon Slump)

0 = No.
1 = Yes, of mild intensity.
2 = Yes, of moderate intensity.
3 = Yes, of severe intensity.

27. Depersonalization/Derealization

0 = Absent.
1 = Mild.
2 = Moderate.
3 = Severe.
4 = Incapacitating.

28. Paranoid Symptoms

0 = None.
1 = Suspicious.
2 = Ideas of reference.
3 = Delusions of reference and persecution.

29. Obsessive/Compulsive

0 = Absent.
1 = Mild.
2 = Severe.

29-item Ham-D Total: _____
(all items)

Patient Health Questionnaire, 9-item version (PHQ-9)

Kroenke K, Spitzer RL, Williams JB. The PHQ-9: validity of a brief depression severity measure. *J Gen Intern Med* 2001; 16:606–613.

Instructions – How to Score the PHQ-9

Major depressive disorder is suggested if:

i. Of the 9 items, 5 or more are checked as at least 'more than half the days'
ii. Either item a. or b. is positive, that is, at least 'more than half the days'

Other depressive syndrome is suggested if:

i. Of the 9 items, a., b. or c. is checked as at least 'more than half the days'
ii. Either item a. or b. is positive, that is, at least 'more than half the days'

Also, PHQ-9 scores can be used to plan and monitor treatment. To score the instrument, tally each response by the number value under the answer headings, (not at all=0, several days=1, more than half the days=2, and nearly every day=3). Add the numbers together to total the score on the bottom of the questionnaire. Interpret the score by using the guide listed below.

Guide for Interpreting PHQ-9 Scores

Score	Recommended Actions
0–4	Normal range or full remission. The score suggests the patient may not need depression treatment.
5–9	Minimal depressive symptoms. Support, educate, call if worse, return in 1 month.
10–14	Major depression, mild severity. Use clinical judgment about treatment, based on patient's duration of symptoms and functional impairment. Treat with antidepressant or psychotherapy.
15–19	Major depression, moderate severity. Warrants treatment for depression, using antidepressant, psychotherapy or a combination of treatment.
20 or higher	Major depression, severe severity. Warrants treatment with antidepressant and psychotherapy, especially if not improved on monotherapy; follow frequently.

Functional Health Assessment

The instrument also includes a functional health assessment. This asks the patient how emotional difficulties or problems impact work, things at home, or relationships with other people. Patient responses can be one of four: Not difficult at all, Somewhat difficult, Very difficult, Extremely difficult. The last two responses suggest that the patient's functionality is impaired. After treatment begins, functional status and number score can be measured to assess patient improvement.

For more information on using the PHQ-9, visit www.depression-primarycare.org

Patient Health Questionnaire (PHQ-9)

Patient name: _____ Date: _ _ _ _ _ _ _

1. Over the last 2 weeks, how often have you been bothered by any of the following problems?

	Not at all (0)	Several days (1)	More than half the days (2)	Nearly every day (3)
a. Little interest or pleasure in doing things.	☐	☐	☐	☐
b. Feeling down, depressed, or hopeless.	☐	☐	☐	☐
c. Trouble falling/staying asleep, sleeping too much.	☐	☐	☐	☐
d. Feeling tired or having little energy.	☐	☐	☐	☐
e. Poor appetite or overeating.	☐	☐	☐	☐
f. Feeling bad about yourself, or that you are a failure, or have let yourself or your family down.	☐	☐	☐	☐
g. Trouble concentrating on things, such as reading the newspaper or watching TV.	☐	☐	☐	☐
h. Moving or speaking so slowly that other people could have noticed. Or the opposite; being so fidgety or restless that you have been moving around more than usual.	☐	☐	☐	☐
i. Thoughts that you would be better off dead or of hurting yourself in some way.	☐	☐	☐	☐

2. If you checked off any problem on this questionnaire so far, how difficult have these problems made it for you to do your work, take care of things at home, or get along with other people?

☐ Not difficult   ☐ Somewhat   ☐ Very   ☐ Extremely
at all   difficult   difficult   difficult

TOTAL SCORE _____

Quick Inventory of Depressive Symptomatology, Self-Rated (QIDS-SR)

Rush AJ, Trivedi MH, Ibrahim HM, Carmody TJ, Arnow B, Klein DN, Markowitz JC, Ninan PT, Kornstein S, Manber R, Thase ME, Kocsis JH, Keller MB. The 16-Item Quick Inventory of Depressive Symptomatology (QIDS), clinician rating (QIDS-C), and self-report (QIDS-SR): a psychometric evaluation in patients with chronic major depression. *Biol Psychiatry* 2003; 54:573–583.

Quick Inventory of Depressive Symptomatology (Self-Report) (QIDS-SR)

NAME: _____ TODAY'S DATE_____

Please circle the one response to each item that best describes you for the past seven days.

1. Falling Asleep:

    0 I never take longer than 30 minutes to fall asleep.
    1 I take at least 30 minutes to fall asleep, less than half the time.
    2 I take at least 30 minutes to fall asleep, more than half the time.
    3 I take more than 60 minutes to fall asleep, more than half the time.

2. Sleep During the Night:

    0 I do not wake up at night.
    1 I have a restless, light sleep with a few brief awakenings each night.
    2 I wake up at least once a night, but I go back to sleep easily.
    3 I awaken more than once a night and stay awake for 20 minutes or more, more than half the time.

3. Waking Up Too Early:

    0 Most of the time, I awaken no more than 30 minutes before I need to get up.
    1 More than half the time, I awaken more than 30 minutes before I need to get up.
    2 I almost always awaken at least one hour or so before I need to, but I go back to sleep eventually.
    3 I awaken at least one hour before I need to, and can't go back to sleep.

4. Sleeping Too Much:

    0 I sleep no longer than 7–8 hours/night, without napping during the day.
    1 I sleep no longer than 10 hours in a 24- hour period including naps.
    2 I sleep no longer than 12 hours in a 24- hour period including naps.
    3 I sleep longer than 12 hours in a 24-hour period including naps.

5. Feeling Sad:

    0 I do not feel sad
    1 I feel sad less than half the time.

2 I feel sad more than half the time.
3 I feel sad nearly all of the time.

6. Decreased Appetite:

    0 There is no change in my usual appetite.
    1 I eat somewhat less often or lesser amounts of food than usual.
    3 I eat much less than usual and only with personal effort.
    4 I rarely eat within a 24-hour period, and only with extreme personal effort or when others persuade me to eat.

7. Increased Appetite:

    0 There is no change from my usual appetite.
    1 I feel a need to eat more frequently than usual.
    2 I regularly eat more often and/or greater amounts of food than usual.
    3 I feel driven to overeat both at mealtime and between meals.

8. Decreased Weight (Within the Last Two Weeks):

    0 I have not had a change in my weight.
    1 I feel as if I've had a slight weight loss.
    2 I have lost 2 pounds or more.
    3 I have lost 5 pounds or more.

9. Increased Weight (Within the Last Two Weeks):

    0 I have not had a change in my weight.
    1 I feel as if I've had a slight weight gain.
    2 I have gained 2 pounds or more.
    3 I have gained 5 pounds or more.

10. Concentration/Decision-Making:

    0 There is no change in my usual capacity to concentrate or make decisions.
    1 I occasionally feel indecisive or find that my attention wanders.
    2 Most of the time, I struggle to focus my attention or to make decisions.

3 I cannot concentrate well enough to read or cannot make even minor decisions.

11.   View of Myself:

0 I see myself as equally worthwhile and deserving as other people.
1 I am more self-blaming than usual.
2 I largely believe that I cause problems for others.
3 I think almost constantly about major and minor defects in myself.

12.   Thoughts of Death or Suicide:

0 I do not think of suicide or death.
1 I feel that life is empty or wonder if it's worth living.
2 I think of suicide or death several times a week for several minutes.
3 I think of suicide or death several times a day in some detail, or I have made specific plans for suicide or have actually tried to take my life.

13.   General Interest:

0 There is no change from usual in how interested I am in other people or activities.
1 I notice that I am less interested in people or activities.
2 I find I have interest in only one or two of my formerly pursued activities.
3 I have virtually no interest in formerly pursued activities.

14.   Energy Level:

0 There is no change in my usual level of energy.
1 I get tired more easily than usual.
2 I have to make a big effort to start or finish my usual daily activities (for example, shopping, homework, cooking or going to work).
3 I really cannot carry out most of my usual daily activities because I just don't have the energy.

15.   Feeling slowed down:

0 I think, speak, and move at my usual rate of speed.
1 I find that my thinking is slowed down or my voice sounds dull or flat.
2 It takes me several seconds to respond to most questions and I'm sure my thinking is slowed.
3 I am often unable to respond to questions without extreme effort.

16.   Feeling restless:

0 I do not feel restless.
1 I'm often fidgety, wringing my hands, or need to shift how I am sitting.
2 I have impulses to move about and am quite restless.
3 At times, I am unable to stay seated and need to pace around.

To Score:

1. Enter the highest score on any 1 of the 4 sleep items (1–4)   _____
2. Item 5   _____
3. Enter the highest score on any 1 appetite/ weight item (6–9)   _____
4. Item 10   _____
5. Item 11   _____
6. Item 12   _____
7. Item 13   _____
8. Item 14   _____
9. Enter the highest score on either of the 2 psychomotor items (15 and 16)   _____

TOTAL SCORE (Range 0–27)   _____

Scoring Criteria	
0–5	Normal
6–10	Mild
11–15	Moderate
16–20	Severe
≥21	Very Severe

Revised 5/1/00

Adverse Events Scale

This is a self-rated scale that we have used in our treatment studies to assess side effects to treatment. It is more detailed than is usually required in clinical practice. However, it can be useful to quantify side effects, especially in people who may be sensitive to them. The scale should be completed by patients at baseline (before treatment) for comparison during treatment.

Adverse Events Scale

Please rate according to these definitions:

- **Slight**: Awareness of a sign or symptom which is easily tolerated.
- **Moderate**: Discomfort enough to cause interference with usual activity.
- **Severe**: Incapacitating with inability to do work or usual activity.

Have you experienced any of the following within the last week or since your last visit?	How troubling or disabling is this for you? Please circle your response.				Do you think this is related to treatment?	
	Not at all	Slight	Moderate	Severe	Yes	No
Anxiety ("feeling wired")	1	2	3	4	Y	N
Nervousness	1	2	3	4	Y	N
Agitation	1	2	3	4	Y	N
Tremor	1	2	3	4	Y	N
Twitching	1	2	3	4	Y	N
Irritability	1	2	3	4	Y	N
Dizziness	1	2	3	4	Y	N
Feeling faint when suddenly standing up	1	2	3	4	Y	N
Tightness in chest	1	2	3	4	Y	N
Palpitations	1	2	3	4	Y	N
Dry mouth	1	2	3	4	Y	N
Abdominal pain	1	2	3	4	Y	N
Heartburn	1	2	3	4	Y	N
Nausea	1	2	3	4	Y	N
Diarrhea	1	2	3	4	Y	N
Constipation	1	2	3	4	Y	N
Sweating	1	2	3	4	Y	N

Flushing	1	2	3	4	Y	N
Swelling	1	2	3	4	Y	N
Muscle pain	1	2	3	4	Y	N
Weakness / fatigue	1	2	3	4	Y	N
Sleepiness	1	2	3	4	Y	N
Decreased appetite	1	2	3	4	Y	N
Increased appetite	1	2	3	4	Y	N
Weight gain	1	2	3	4	Y	N
Weight loss	1	2	3	4	Y	N
Increased sleep	1	2	3	4	Y	N
Decreased sleep	1	2	3	4	Y	N
Sleep disturbance	1	2	3	4	Y	N
Headache	1	2	3	4	Y	N
Blurred vision	1	2	3	4	Y	N
Other eye or vision problems	1	2	3	4	Y	N
Rash	1	2	3	4	Y	N
Increased sex drive	1	2	3	4	Y	N
Decreased sex drive	1	2	3	4	Y	N
Male erection problems	1	2	3	4	Y	N
Female lubrication problems	1	2	3	4	Y	N
Delayed orgasm	1	2	3	4	Y	N
Spontaneous orgasm	1	2	3	4	Y	N
Premature ejaculation	1	2	3	4	Y	N
Delayed ejaculation	1	2	3	4	Y	N

Sample insurance reimbursement letter

This is a sample letter that we have used for patients seeking reimbursement for light devices from their health insurance company. Many companies have approved reimbursement on a case-by-case basis, so documentation by the health practitioner can be helpful.

To whom it may concern:

Seasonal affective disorder (SAD), or winter clinical depression, is an accepted psychiatric diagnosis with standardized diagnostic criteria. In the most recent edition of the Diagnostic and Statistical Manual of Mental Disorders (DSM-IV-TR), the standard medical classification system published by the American Psychiatric Association, SAD is listed as a *seasonal pattern* course specifier for:

CODE NO.	DIAGNOSIS
DSM-IV-296.3x	Major Depressive Disorder, Recurrent
DSM-IV-296.4x	Bipolar Disorder, Manic
DSM-IV-296.5x	Bipolar Disorder, Depressed
DSM-IV-296.6x	Bipolar Disorder, Mixed
DSM-IV-296.70	Bipolar Disorder, NOS

The current recommended first-line treatment for SAD or *seasonal pattern* is light therapy. Light therapy is now a standard medical treatment and is no longer considered experimental. Light therapy has been included as a recommended treatment for SAD in the latest clinical practice guidelines of the American Psychiatric Association, the Canadian Psychiatric Association, the World Federation of Societies of Biological Psychiatry, and other agencies. Summary references for these clinical guidelines are included below.

In order to administer light therapy, a 10,000 lux fluorescent light box or other light device is required. This light box and treatment should be regarded as a medical necessity and preferable to other forms of treatment.

Sincerely,

PRACTITIONER NAME
Practitioner Address

References

American Psychiatric Association. Practice Guideline for the Treatment of Patients with Major Depressive Disorder (Revision, April, 2000). *American Journal of Psychiatry*, Vol. 157, No.4 (Supplement), p. 31, 2000. www.psych.org

Bauer M, Whybrow PC, Angst J. Versiani M, Moller H-J. World Federation of Societies of Biological Psychiatry (WFSBP) guidelines for biological treatment of unipolar depressive disorders, Part 1: Acute and continuation treatment of major depressive disorder. *World Journal of Biological Psychiatry*, Vol. 3, pp. 5–43, 2002.

Kennedy SH, Lam RW, Cohen NL, Ravindran AV. Clinical guidelines for the treatment of depressive disorders. IV. Pharmacotherapy and other biological treatments. *Canadian Journal of Psychiatry*, Vol. 46, Supplement 1, pp. 38S-58S, 2001. www.cpa-apc.org

Lam RW, Levitt AJ. (editors). *Canadian Consensus Guidelines for the Treatment of Seasonal Affective Disorder*. Vancouver, BC; Clinical & Academic Publishing, 1999, ISBN 0-9685874-0-2. Available at www.UBCsad.ca

INDEX